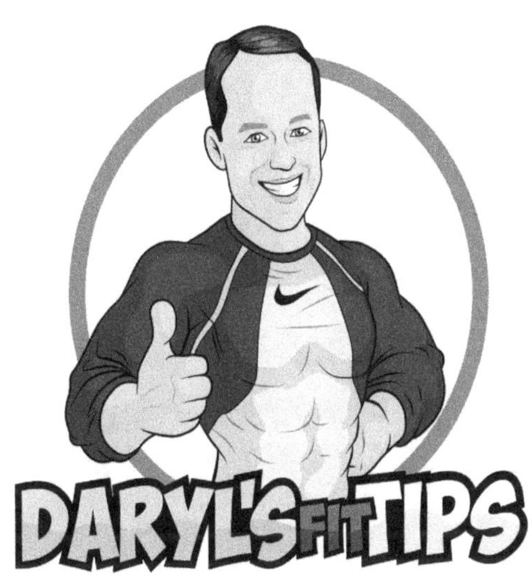

100 Great Nutrition and Fitness Tips

Volume TWO

Daryl Conant, M.Ed.

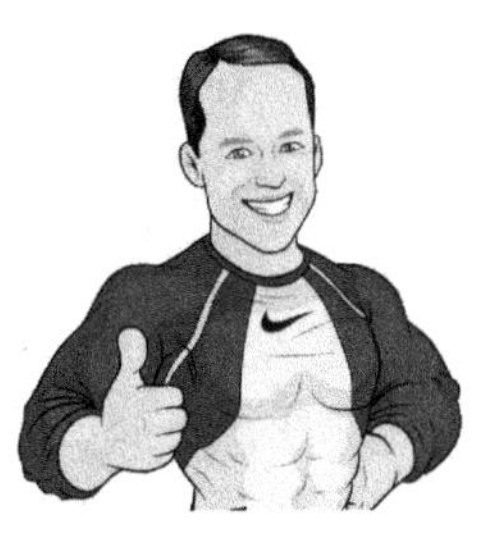

Daryl's FIT TIPS

Volume II

2018

Disclaimer

The content displayed in Daryl's FIT TIPS including blog posts, articles, videos, tip, and testimonials are my personal beliefs and are meant for informational purposes only. These tips, opinions, and writings are not intended to diagnose, treat, or cure any health problems. In addition, this information is not meant to replace your doctor's recommendations or the advice of other qualified healthcare professionals. Always check with your doctor before beginning a new fitness or nutrition program.

To the best of my knowledge, the information provided within Healthy Living is believed to be true and accurate; however, the reader should assume all responsibility for consulting with his/her doctor regarding any health matter. Daryl Conant denies any liability, loss, or injury in relationship with any opinion, tip, or exercise shared is this publication.

Daryl Conant, M.Ed.

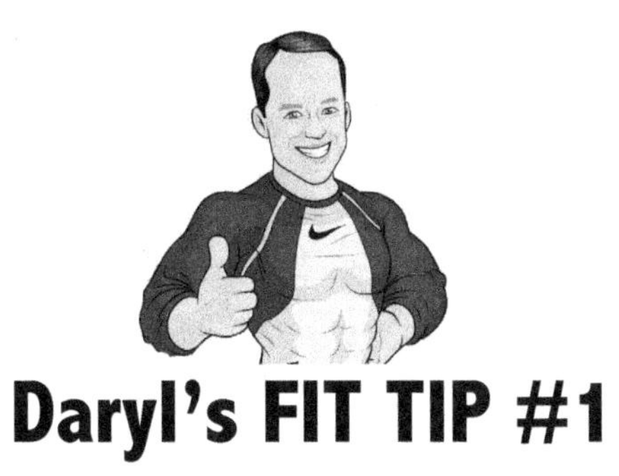

Daryl's FIT TIP #1

YOUR BRAIN

The brain is the control center of the body. A poor functioning brain results in a plethora of neurophysiological issues.

I am convinced that the majority of brain dysfunction is directly related to toxic nutrition and chemical compounds (drugs, pesticides, herbicides, additives, etc.) that people are exposed to every day.

All of the systems of the body work together in unison, if one system is compromised then the entire physiological chain is affected.

Toxic food and drugs destroy the digestive properties of the intestines, which will produce a firestorm of enzymatic chaos, resulting in adverse effects on health. For example, obesity is a side effect of a dysfunctional metabolic pathway.

In order to heal the body, the root of the problem must be resolved. Simply taking drugs, or removing organs from the body is not always the best solution and should be used only in life and death scenarios.

The entire physiological spectrum of the body must be taken into consideration when dealing with poor health issues.

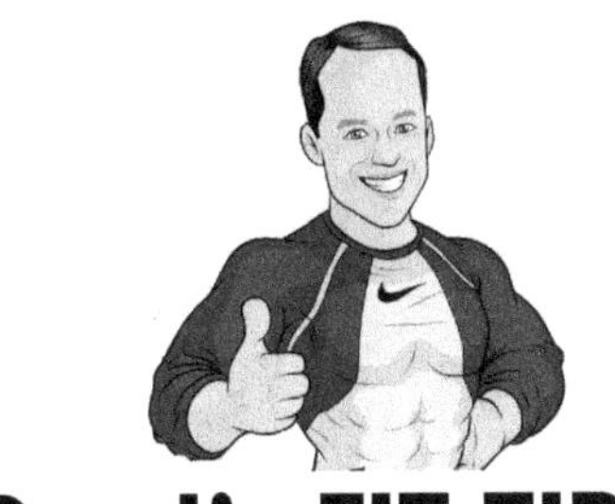

Daryl's FIT TIP #2

UP YOURS!

If you are tired of being tired then it's time to increase your energy. Consistent exercise and eating a wholesome balanced diet rich in healthy fats will increase and improve the production of the mitochondria of muscle cells. The mitochondria is the powerhouse of the cell and is where the high energy phosphate compound (ATP) is produced.

High levels of ATP provide the body with an enormous amount of energy. This is why little kids can go on and on without ever getting tired, they are producing ATP at an incredibly fast rate. ATP levels wane as people get older, especially if the person doesn't eat a healthy diet or exercise.

Sustained aerobic exercise for 15-30 minutes a day can boost the mitochondria and yield a ton of ATP. So UP YOURS by building and utilizing the incredible ability of the mitochondria.

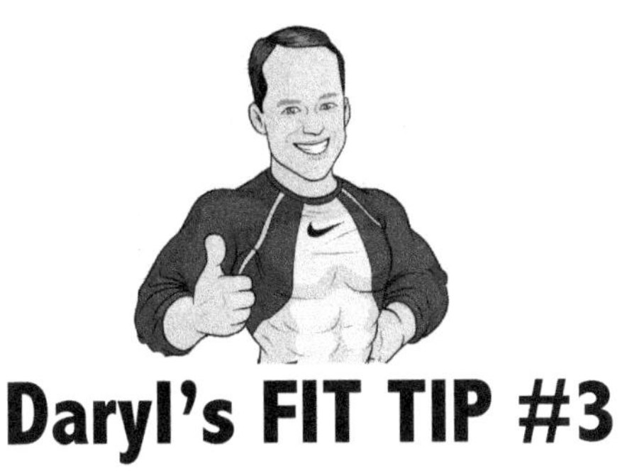

Daryl's FIT TIP #3

TIGHT CLOTHES

Wearing tight clothes all the time can increase musculoskeletal dysfunction (back, hips, shoulders, etc.). The tight clothes restrict the range of motion of a particular joint reducing muscle extensibility.

If the person has to make a quick bending or reaching movement the clothes can limit the range of motion, which could displace undue stress in other areas of the body, i.e. lower back.

Not being able to bend over efficiently can compromise the lower back musculature because the person's legs remain locked when the person bends over.

Even though tight clothes look great on folks that have a "hot" body, they could result in musculoskeletal dysfunction.

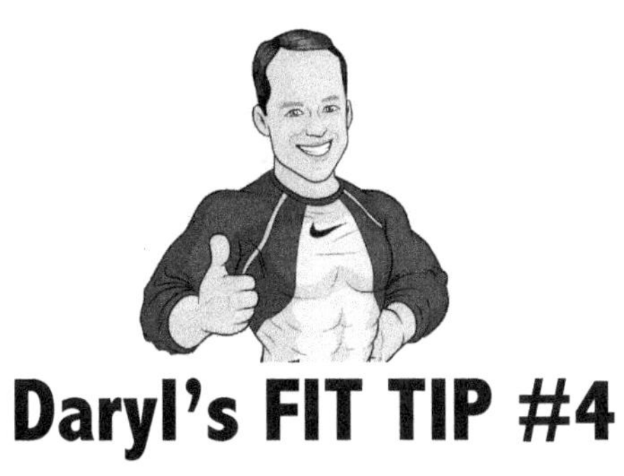

Daryl's FIT TIP #4

THE GLUTEN FAD-DIET TRAP

Millions of people have cut gluten to lose weight, gain energy and/or reduce gastrointestinal distress after eating. Contrary to popular belief, however, gluten-free does not equal healthy.

Only 1% of the population has celiac disease. Everyone else has fallen into the fad-diet trap. It is believed that people are "healed" by removing gluten from their diet, but it is not a magical cure. They are simply removing the bread, chips, cookies, pastries, grains, and high sugary snacks from their diet. Of course when you eliminate these foods you will see a difference in your health and body composition.

Gluten that has not been tampered with has no effect on a person who doesn't have celiac disease. So instead of eliminating gluten, replace your simple carbohydrates with complex carbs from vegetables, beans, legumes, and non-GMO-whole grains. Choose brown rice instead of white rice.

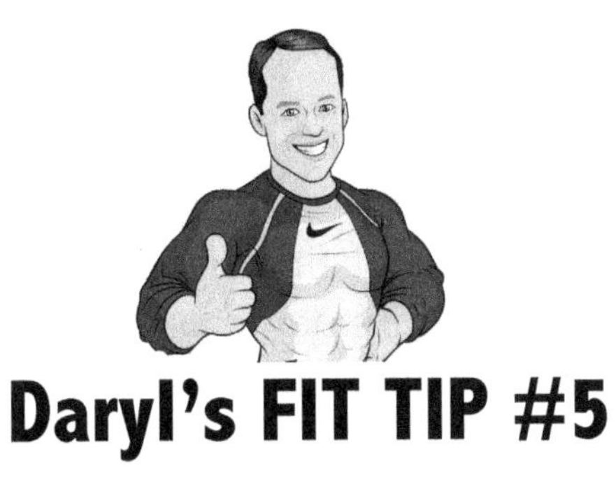

Daryl's FIT TIP #5

EVEN THOUGH

Even though a person eats healthy nutrient dense foods and abstains from junk food doesn't necessarily mean that they will lose body fat while maintaining or increasing lean body tissue (i.e., muscle).

Not knowing what your daily nutrient requirement is based on your own metabolism, body composition, and energy output, will hinder your progress. So many folks have no idea what their daily nutrient requirement is, they follow the silly calorie myth to determine how much food to consume.

Eating one egg, a spear of organic broccoli, a handful of organic nuts, and an organic yogurt per day is not going to be enough to sustain your metabolic demand, which will result in muscle wasting and fat storage.

Having your metabolism tested is one of the most accurate ways of finding out what your daily nutrient requirement is. By increasing or decreasing your nutrient intake can dramatically change your fat burning metabolism.

It's not about EXERCISING MORE and EATING LESS, it's about knowing exactly how many nutrients you need per day to feed the vital nutrient exchange system of the body and to stay in FAT METABOLISM, burning fat all day long.

If you are interested in having your metabolism tested please message me and I will give you more information.

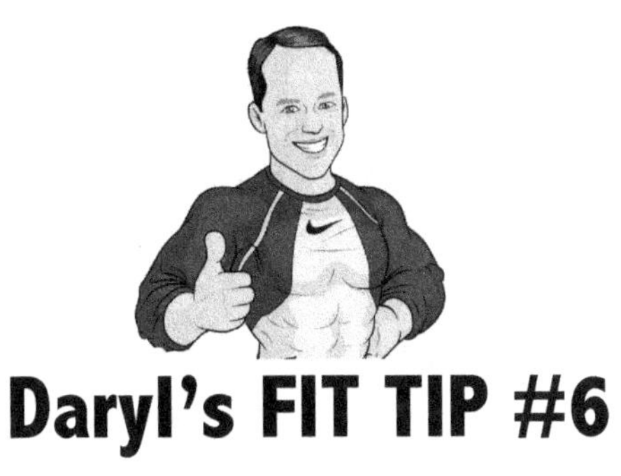

Daryl's FIT TIP #6

POSITOPES

Avoid all the negitopes within the mass of collective energy and collect as many POSITOPES as possible to enrich your stream of consciousness with a surge of positive energy.

Every second of the day we collect and process external information through touch, taste, smell, sight, and hearing. The information gets processed and encoded in our stream of consciousness and compartmentalized into the various brain centers. The energy derived from this process is the energy that you become.

Constantly being influenced by negitopes (negative stimuli) will produce a negative energy flow in the body compromising good health. By constantly striving to absorb and process positopes (all things positive) the body will become charged with positive energy. This positive energy will then emit from your own body and you will become a positopic energy source yourself, therefore attracting others like you.

Stay away from all the negitopes, they are TOXIC to your health. Collect and surround yourself with POSITOPES and see how your health and attitude will change.

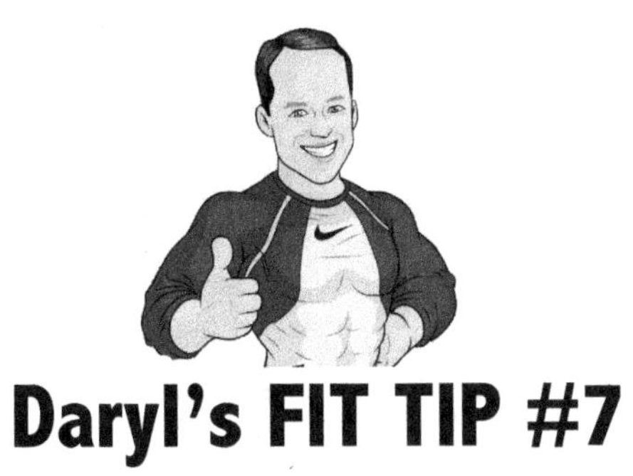

Daryl's FIT TIP #7

MUSCLE GROWTH

Muscle growth occurs whenever the rate of muscle protein synthesis is greater than the rate of muscle protein breakdown.

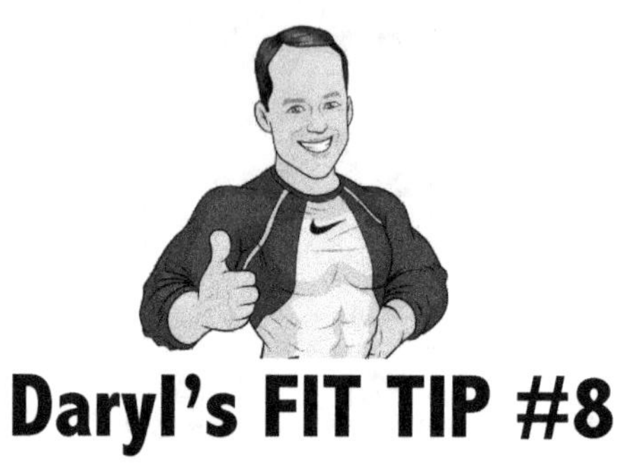

Daryl's FIT TIP #8

CONNECTED

Everything that we see, taste, smell, hear, touch, and think about gets transferred and processed in our body every day. If the stimulus is negative the body will shift into a negative state, compromising the immune system and homeostasis. One negative side effect is tissue breakdown and fat storage. The cells become weaker and less powerful in a negative state.

If the stimulus is positive the opposite effect occurs, the body becomes charged with positive energy making the cells energized.

Collect as many positopes during the day as you can and watch your health improve dramatically.

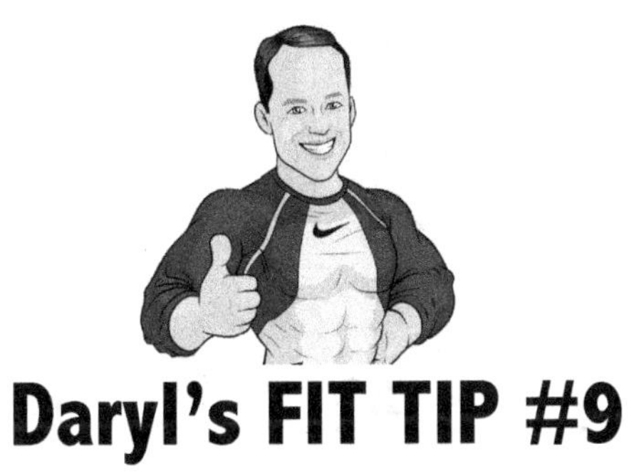

Daryl's FIT TIP #9

ONE REASON

One reason why people can't seem to heal their metabolism and reduce BODY FAT is because they are UNWILLING to follow the parameters of basic physiology.

Some people are reluctant to ever remove the causes to the problem. Instead, they will try to fix the problem by seeking out the "magic pill" approach, this will NEVER work.

OBESITY is a side effect of a dysfunctional metabolism. Heal the metabolism, reduce the fat.

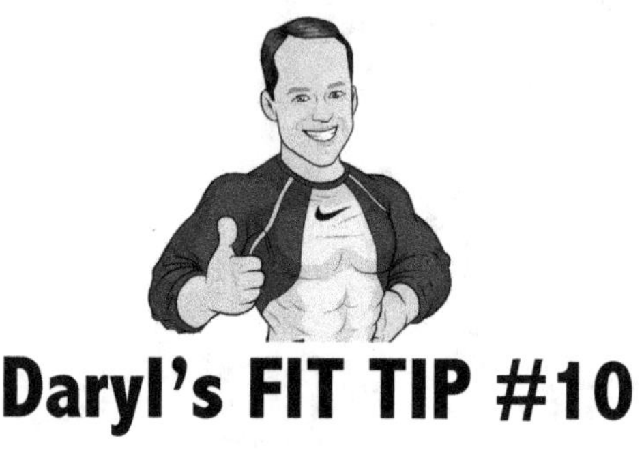

Daryl's FIT TIP #10

OVER FAT

Excess body fat beyond your set point indicates an abnormal shift in the metabolic pathways of the body. In order to resolve the excess fat problem, the dysfunction within the metabolism MUST be fixed.

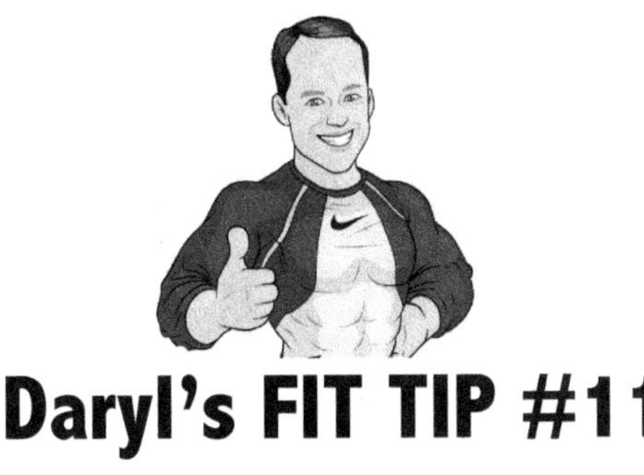

Daryl's FIT TIP #11

FORCEFUL CONTRACTIONS

It is important to always create a forceful contraction of the muscle. Poor contraction indicates weak nerve synapses, which will result in no gains. A strong contraction will activate a greater neuronal response and pull more blood into the muscle, producing a stronger synaptic transmission and resulting in better gains.

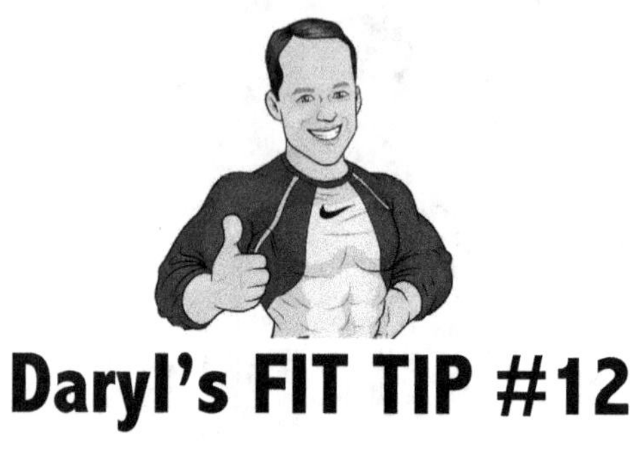

Daryl's FIT TIP #12

Be YOUR BEST

Be the best version of you for your age.

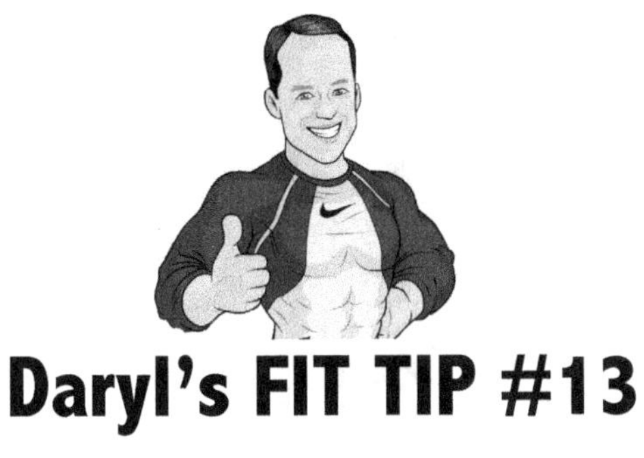

Daryl's FIT TIP #13

DEGENERATIVE DISEASE

Degenerative diseases are NOT genetic but acquired. Because the systems of the human body are interconnected and because one imbalance creates another imbalance, POOR EATING and LIFESTYLE HABITS, not genetics, are the cause of degenerative disease.

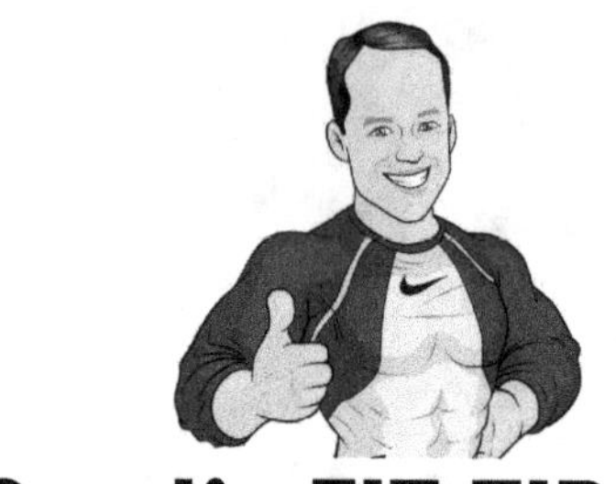

Daryl's FIT TIP #14

IMBALANCE

I have found that there is no significant advantage to performing single arm lifting movements like a one arm chest press or a one arm shoulder press. I feel that performing such exercises with heavy weight will displace the correct biomechanical balance, which could result in injury. It is better to hold two dumbbells and then lift one arm through the range of motion, while the other arm is stabilizing the body.

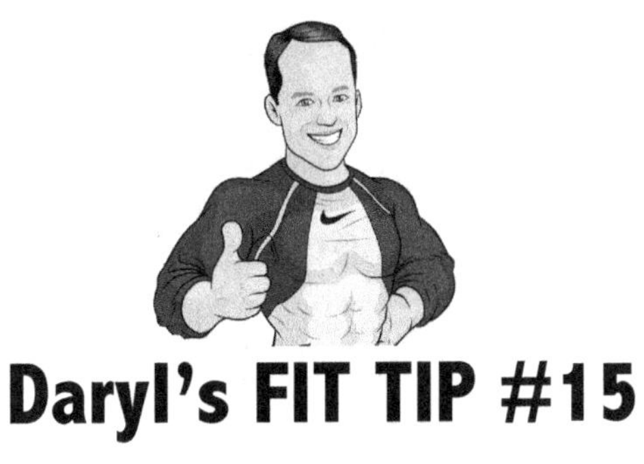

Daryl's FIT TIP #15

HOW MUCH PROTEIN

I am often asked the question, "How much protein should I consume per day?" This is not a one-line answer. There are many variables to consider. However, rather than getting into all of the different variables, I will give you some suggestions.

1. Make sure to take in good organic REAL protein sources that provide a COMPLETE protein profile, meaning they should have both essential and non-essential amino acids.

2. Don't get bogged down with numbers. The average intake of complete protein is about .60% x your lean body mass. If you are sedentary, this value would be .40% x your lean body mass. These numbers are just estimates. They will vary from person to person depending on their genetic profile,

bone structure, body composition, and activity level.

3. There is no need to over-consume protein. Taking in hundreds of grams of protein per day is not going to get you to your goal quicker, in fact, it could hinder your progress.

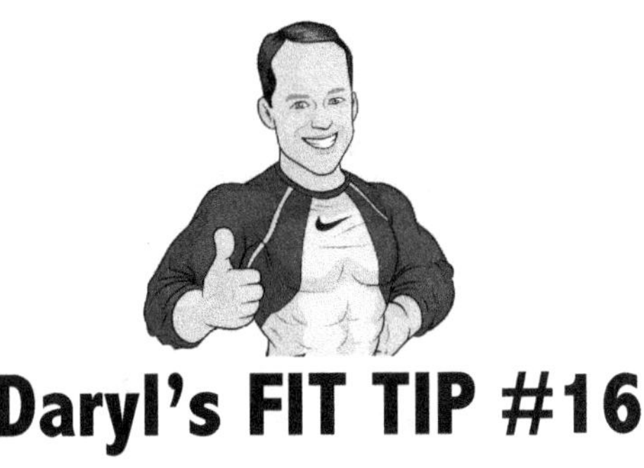

Daryl's FIT TIP #16

LEMON-ZEST

Squeeze fresh lemon into your water to reap the benefits of a natural detoxing drink. Lemon contains Citrate, which is a naturally-occurring inhibitor of toxins in the body. Citrate helps flush out the crystallized toxins. Toxins come into our systems through various sources from the air we breathe to some of the foods we eat. Lemons also contain hesperidin (a citrus bioflavonoid) that helps protect the liver from damage. Also, lemon water helps with digestion and absorption of nutrients. So, I suggest that you drink lemon water after your dinner to help enhance the body's enzyme function and to stimulate the liver.

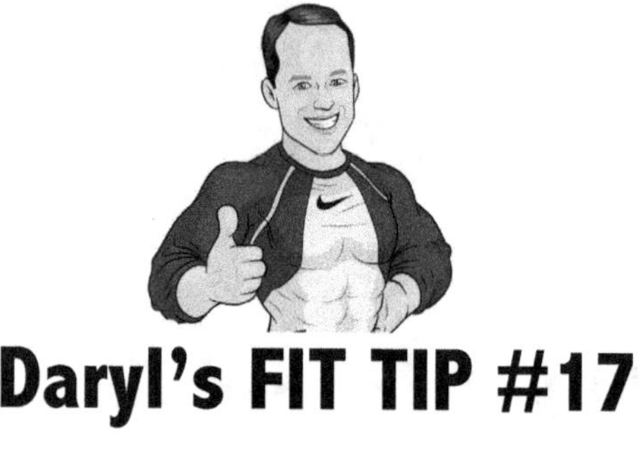

Daryl's FIT TIP #17

GENETIC ABNORMALITY

I believe that the increase in genetic abnormalities (i.e., altered fat genes) over the past 70 years are directly linked to the influence of toxic nutrition and environmental biochemicals.

Toxic nutrition alters the genetic codes of the body causing the physiological systems of the body to create new pathways to try and balance homeostasis, which then leads to the overproduction of various hormones, glucose, fats, and proteins resulting in a variety of different metabolic abnormalities.

This is why there are so many drugs being produced today. Drug companies are trying to keep up with all of the metabolic abnormalities that are constantly developing.

I feel that the more exposure to these toxic compounds moving forward into the future will forever change the evolutionary genomes of the human species, therefore producing many different mutated forms of the HUMAN BEING.

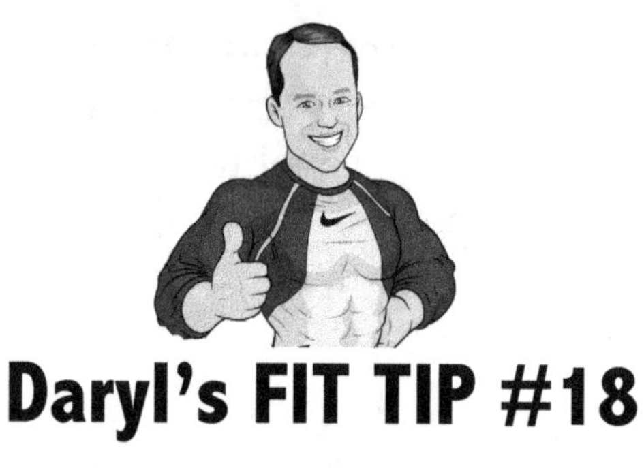

Daryl's FIT TIP #18

WEIGHT DISTRIBUTION

Where you distribute weight on your body is an indication of different metabolic processes.

To resolve the FAT gain issue it is important to FIX the dysfunctional event occurring in the metabolic chain. Not knowing how to resolve the issue properly can result in GREATER WEIGHT GAIN or further physiological dysfunction.

Remember: Exercising more and eating less doesn't always work... This could actually make you FATTER.

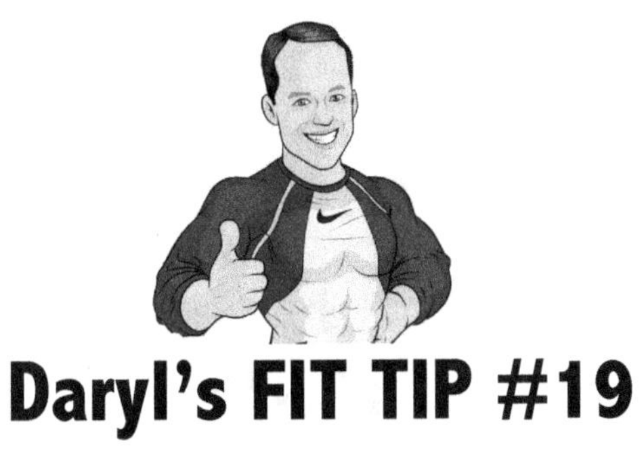

Daryl's FIT TIP #19

CAN YOU GUESS IT

Can you guess what super-food this is?

It contains the following nutrients:
Vitamin A, D, E, K2,F
Lauric Acid: Anti-cancer
Lecithin: an anecdote to cholesterol
Selenium
Iodine
Omega 3
MCT- Medium Chained Triglycerides

Answer: butter

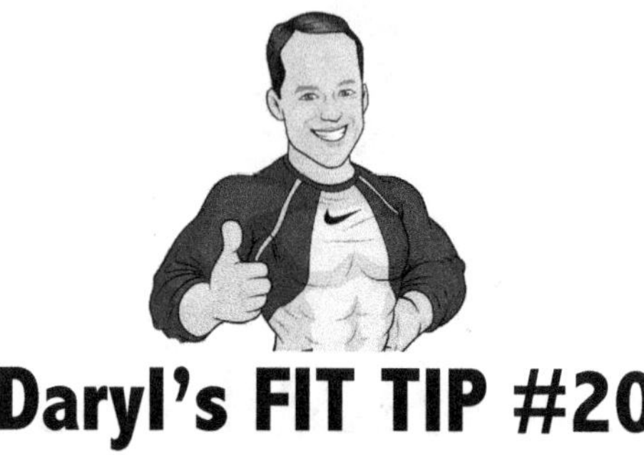

Daryl's FIT TIP #20

A SIMPLE SOLUTION

Folks who consume chocolate, coffee, peppermint, tomato products and alcoholic beverages on a regular basis tend to develop heartburn (acid reflux). In fact, 60 millon Americans per month suffer from this problem. However, there is a simple solution, STOP consuming these products. By doing so will help restore the natural acidic pH balance of the stomach.

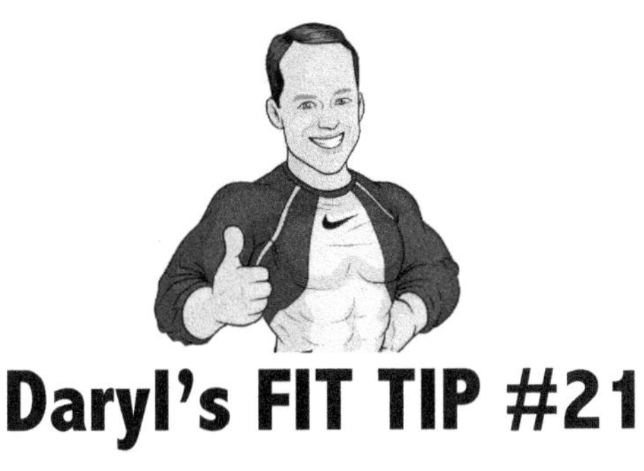

Daryl's FIT TIP #21

STOP SHRINKAGE

The aging body naturally shrinks (atrophy). The most noticeable sign is in skeletal muscle. Skeletal muscle loses its protein suspension and reduces in size (sarcopenia). This is due to a lower concentration of the body's natural anabolic hormones. BUT DON'T FRET, there is a way to slow down the shrinking of the muscles.

Resistance training is the BEST way to maintain skeletal muscle. As long as the body realizes that it is still be challenged by resistive forces it will continue to produce the anabolic properties necessary to keep up with the metabolic demand of the muscle tissue.

Even though sarcopenia will still develop with the aging body you can significantly reduce the speed at which it occurs through weight training methods.

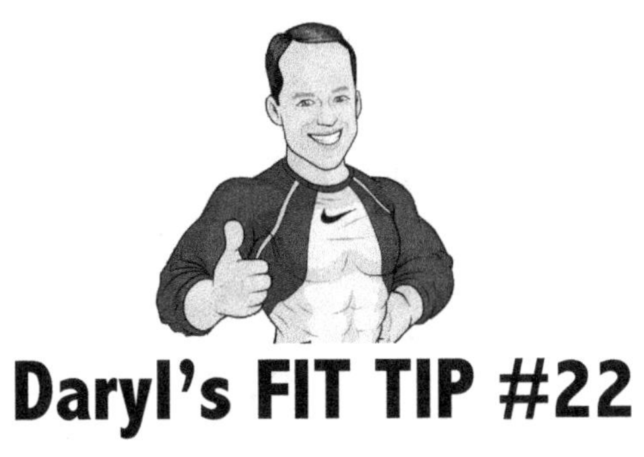

Daryl's FIT TIP #22

HAIL TO SUNSHINE

Vitamin D is one of the keys to getting calcium to your bones, where it belongs. By simply exposing your skin to the sun for about 5-10 minutes 2 to 3 times per week is all you need to get your recommended dose of Vitamin D.

Another benefit from the sun is the closer it is to the earth from May to September the higher the body's natural level of serotonin. Serotonin is a neurotransmitter that helps regulate the brain and central nervous system.

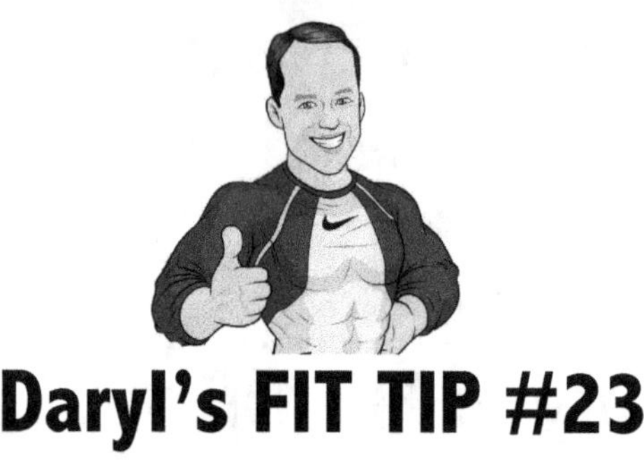

Daryl's FIT TIP #23

HAPPINESS

There can be no health without HAPPINESS. Learn how to live a well-balanced life and reach your potential inner peace. Seek out as many POSITOPES as you can during the day, doing so will charge your body with a high level of positive energy.

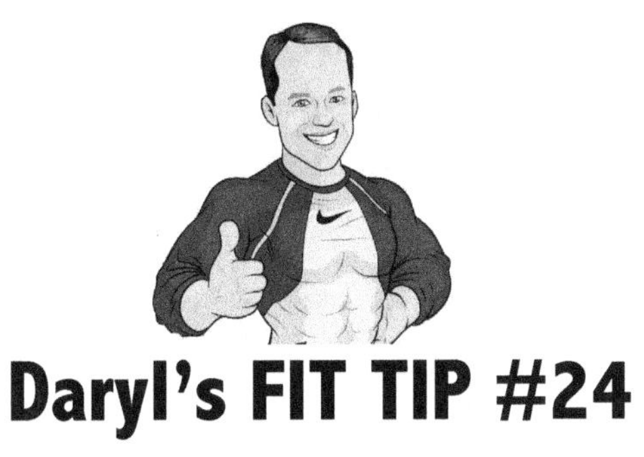

Daryl's FIT TIP #24

REPETITIVE TRAUMA

There is nothing more debilitating than back pain. Chronic pain increases the body's inflammatory processes, which in turn can reduce serotonin levels resulting in irritability and depression making the pain even greater. Back pain is developed through chronic repetitive trauma, lower crossed syndrome, and upper crossed syndrome. There are 3 mistakes that folks make when dealing with back pain.

1. Stretching the wrong muscles to alleviate the pain. In some cases, stretching can make the condition worse.

2. Doing the wrong exercises to work the back can also be problematic.

3. Resting or avoiding exercise to fix the problem. This also is the wrong approach because the supporting muscles become weaker making the situation worse.

To FIX back pain it is important to understand the proper biomechanical kinetic links associated with the anterior and posterior chains. Most of the time back pain is associated with improper biomechanical posture, weak appendicular musculature, or imbalanced muscle development (i.e., overpowering quadricep muscles compared to weaker hamstrings).

If you live in the Kennebunk, Maine area and suffer from back pain drop by my gym and I will give you a FREE evaluation to determine the right procedures to follow to help you.

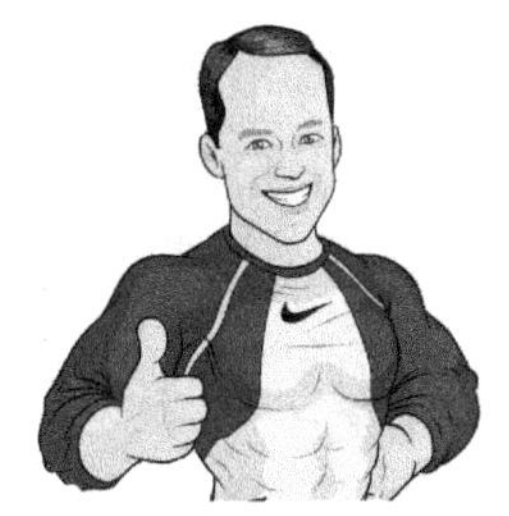

Daryl's FIT TIP #25

7 STEPS TO KEEPING BLOOD PRESSURE IN CHECK

1. Slash the salt. Salt makes your kidneys hold water putting more pressure on your artery walls.

2. Fat midsection. Extra fat around the waist increases blood pressure.

3. Move more. Cardiovascular exercise helps improve the strength and integrity of the lungs, heart, and arteries.

4. Eat more potassium. Potassium lowers sodium. Foods rich in potassium are: avocados, spinach, broccoli.

5. Quit smoking. Nothing good comes from smoking.

6. Calm down. Stress can raise blood pressure.

7. Cut down sugar consumption. Too much sugar wrecks havoc in the body; weakens arteries, increases blood pressure, increases inflammation, increases cholesterol levels, increases fat storage, and increases the growth of bad intestinal bacteria.

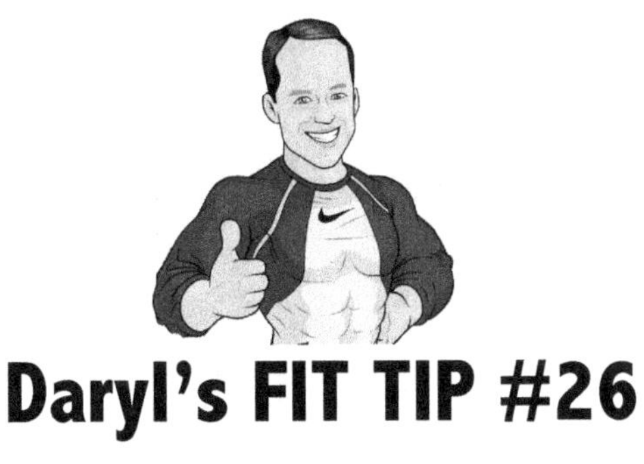

Daryl's FIT TIP #26

FREE YOUR MIND

The brain has a way of carving out its own downtime, characterized by what is called the "default-mode network"-- basically, brain activity that takes place when you're daydreaming or keeping your mind blank. So put away the smartphone for 15 minutes a day and let your brain idle. It will pay dividends in better brain functioning.

.

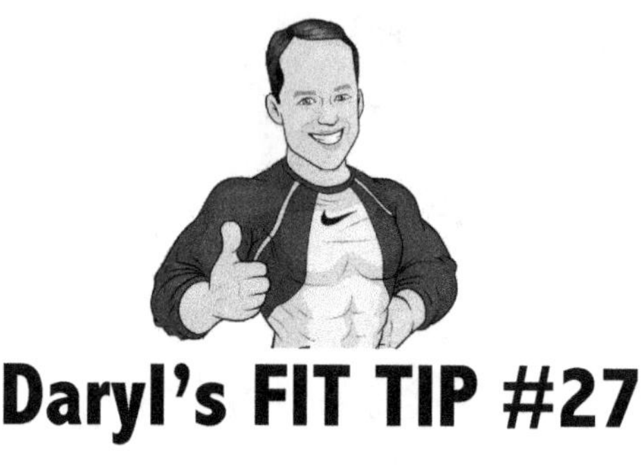

Daryl's FIT TIP #27

ALTOGETHER NOW

Studies have shown that exercise performed in a group-- such as playing a team sport or taking part in one of FNH's awesome fitness classes-- promotes the production of oxytocin, the hormone commonly held responsible for bonding with others. Some evidence has shown close friendships lead to a lower risk for heart problems, so take advantage of your gym's group classes and feel the love start to flow.

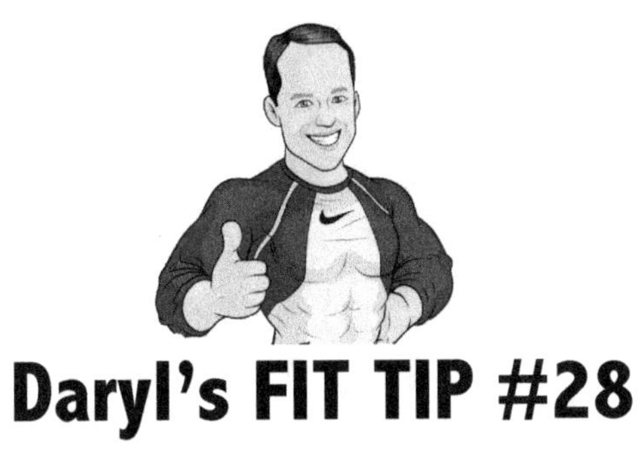

Daryl's FIT TIP #28

5 KEYS To HEALTH and HEALING

1. Proper Nerve Supply. If nerves are blocked or pinched the target tissue can't function properly.

2. Regular Exercise. Movement helps the body regenerate itself and boosts immunity.

3. Proper Nutrition. Nutrient dense foods are the essence of life.

4. Sufficient Rest. Sleep restores and rebuilds the body.

5. Prayer and Meditation. Tranquility calms the nervous system and allows healing and homeostasis.

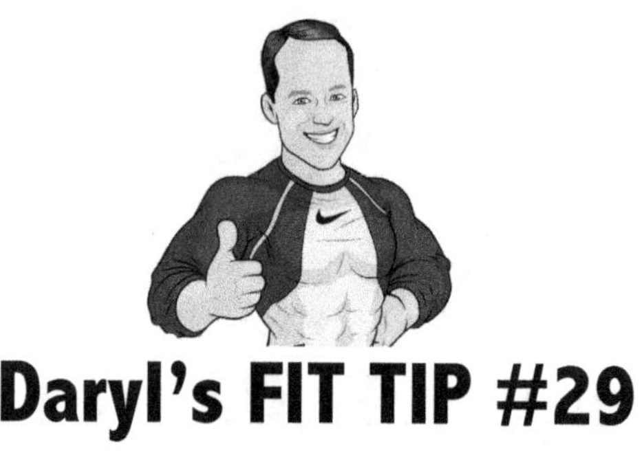

Daryl's FIT TIP #29

KNOW THY PEE

Your urine can tell you a lot about your hydration level.

Symptoms of DEHYDRATION include:
* Little or no urine, or urine that is darker than usual
* Dry mouth
* Sleepiness or fatigue
* Extreme thirst
* Headache
* Confusion
* Feeling dizzy or light-headed
* No tears when crying
* Constipation
* Muscle Cramping

If you are dehydrated it could mean more:
DANGER ZONE:
May indicate kidney disease or liver disease.

Drink early. Don't wait for thirst to hit. By the time you feel the urge to hoist a glass, you're already on your way to dehydration. Thirst only hits after two or more cups of total body water have been lost.

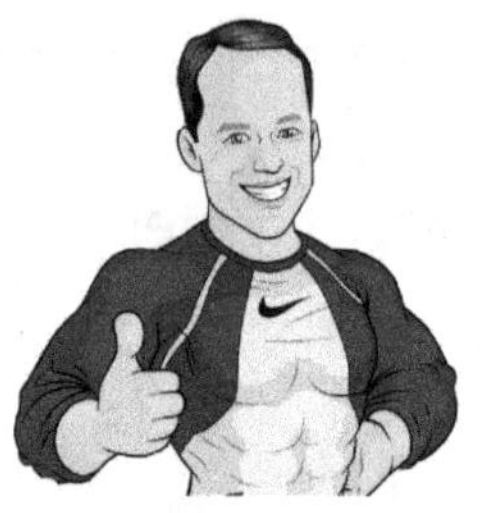

Daryl's FIT TIP #30

EXERCISE CAN MAKE YOU SMARTER

You can think of fitness training as changing the molecular and cellular building blocks that underlie many cognitive skills.

Exercise stimulates the creation of new neurons in the region of the hippocampus that files away experience and new knowledge.

Exercise stimulates the production of new synapses, the connections that constitute functional circuits and whose capacity and efficiency underlie superior intelligence.

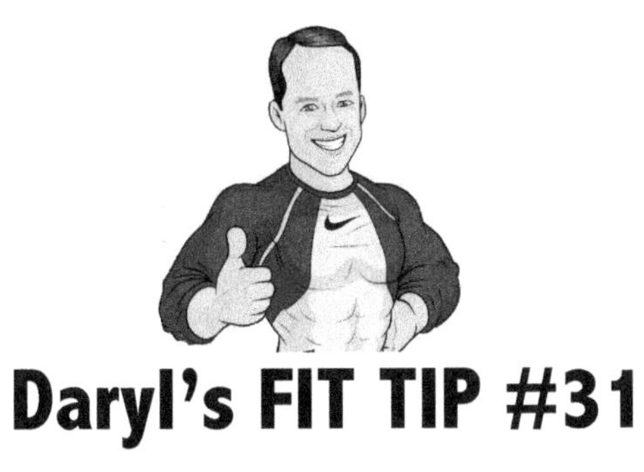

Daryl's FIT TIP #31

FACTS ON GAS

Your digestive gas is made up of mostly nitrogen, hydrogen, and carbon dioxide, with a little oxygen and occasionally some methane. Gas and bloating occur when carbohydrates undigested by the small intestine ferment in the colon, causing the most recognizable (and least convenient) side effect of gas: the dreaded FART.

An occasional release is normal and sometimes welcomed among sophomoric kinship where the lighting of the eternal flame can bring hours of amusement, but chronic gas can indicate a health problem. Excess gas and bloating may be a symptom of IBS, Chron's disease, ulcerative colitis, or diabetes.

To help reduce the gas build up in the intestines I recommend that you exercise. Physical activity helps target the muscles that help move food and gas through your system more efficiently. It also helps to eat smaller, more frequent meals, which are easier for your body to break down. And, avoid or limit your intake of gas-producing foods, i.e., certain fruits, beans, starchy vegetables.

This fit tip STINKS... ha, ha, ha...

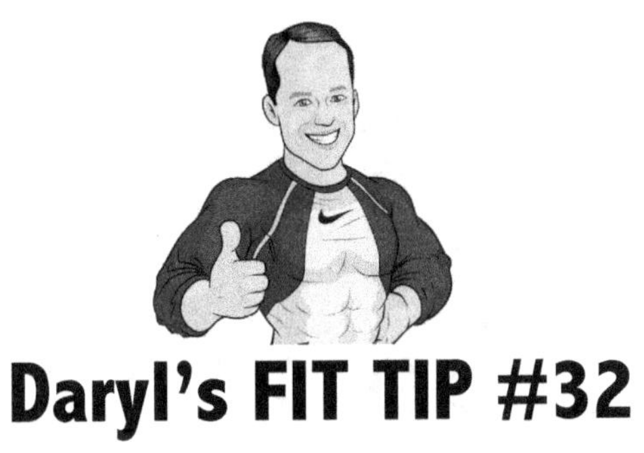

Daryl's FIT TIP #32

NATURAL HIGH

A study released earlier this year indicates school children who are regularly exposed to nature perform better on cognition tests of memories. For adults, a study has shown that nature walks help reduce activity in the part of your brain associated with ruminative, self-destructive thoughts. So get out in the greenery for your own good.

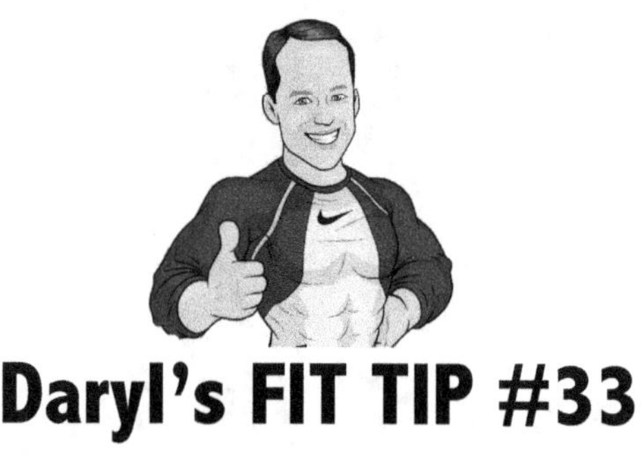

Daryl's FIT TIP #33

NUTS and SEED

A significant source of vitamin E, nuts, almonds, cashews, peanuts, sunflower seeds, sesame seeds, flaxseed and unhydrogenated nut butters such as, peanut butter, almond butter and tahini are a smart, healthy snack.

Vitamin E protects the brain's iron from exposure to oxygen, which breaks down the brain-- think of a rusting piece of metal-- and increases the risk of diseases including Alzheimer's and cancer. Vitamin E also helps quench free radicals, which can destabilize the brain.

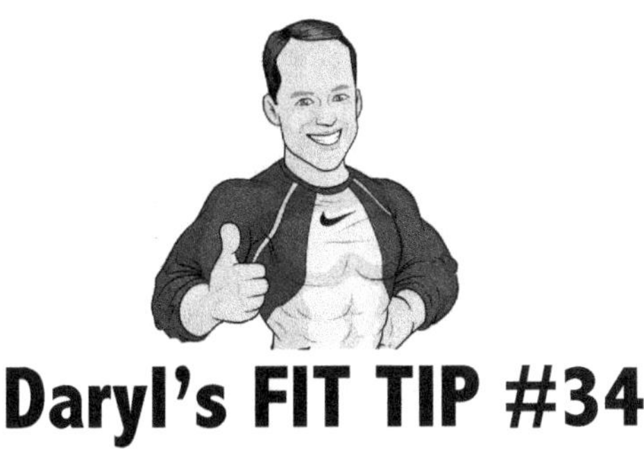

Daryl's FIT TIP #34

CONNECTED

There can be no health without HAPPINESS.

The body has 6 senses: taste, sight, hearing, touch, smell, and intuition. In order to stay healthy, all of the senses must be stimulated in a POSITIVE way to keep the physiological balance of the body working efficiently. If a sense is influenced by negative energy then the entire synergy of the cellular network is compromised. The brain deciphers all of the information being collected by the senses and then relays the information through a vast neuronal network.

Depending on the information received will determine what hormone or hormones are released. If the information received is negative then stress chemicals will be released to defend the body. If the information is positive then the body will release healing chemicals that will boost immunity and health.

The GOAL for life is to collect as MANY POSITOPES as you can every day to supercharge your physiological systems.

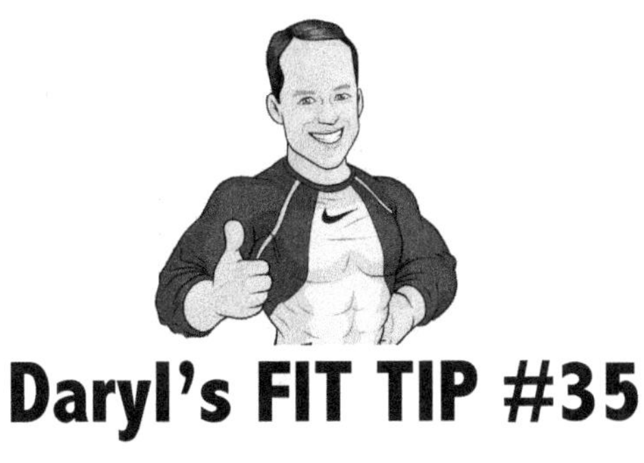

Daryl's FIT TIP #35

A PUZZLING THOUGHT

A new study suggests those who read, write and do crosswords or other puzzles throughout their lives have a significant less beta-amyloid protein, a major component of the brain plaque that's a marker of Alzheimer's disease.

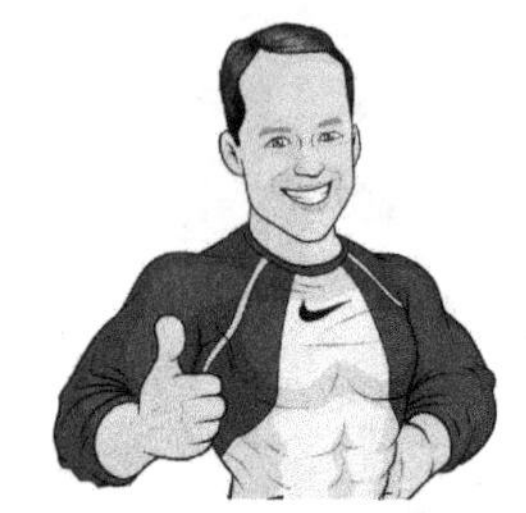

Daryl's FIT TIP #36

STOP THE WORRY CYCLE

Your hormones can get out of kilter when you're stressed, tired or eating poorly, creating tons of trouble for your body---which creates more stress. Physical activity, especially resistance, releases hormones such as serotonin, cortisol, and androgen that stabilize your disposition.

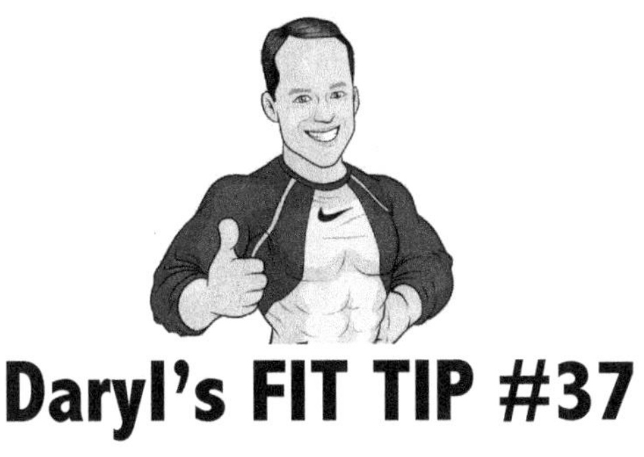

Daryl's FIT TIP #37

YOUR BODY

From the rush of a good workout to the embrace of a loved one, you only have one body through which to experience the joys of living. Better take care of it!

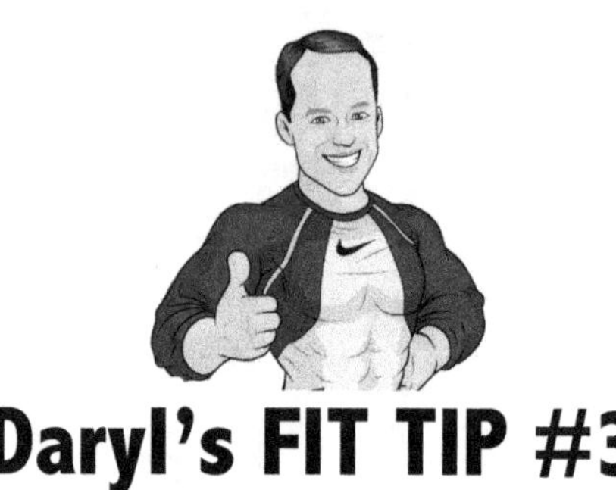

Daryl's FIT TIP #38

LYME DISEASE

Lyme disease was extremely rare before the industrial age. This is because most folks living in rural areas had a small farm where they had their own chickens roaming free in the yard. Chickens eat ticks. As industry expanded folks had to travel further for work leaving behind the farm. Eventually, small farms would decrease significantly in number, allowing an insurgence of ticks.

Today, Lyme disease is an epidemic in America. It is not realistic to think that everyone can have chickens running around the yard these days, but there is a safe way to divert ticks from crawling up your leg. Diane Emery from the gym suggests that rubbing Vicks Vapor Rub on your shoes can help keep ticks off. Apparently, ticks can't stand the smell of Vicks Vapor Rub. Vicks Vapor Rub is a safer alternative to some of the tick sprays out there.

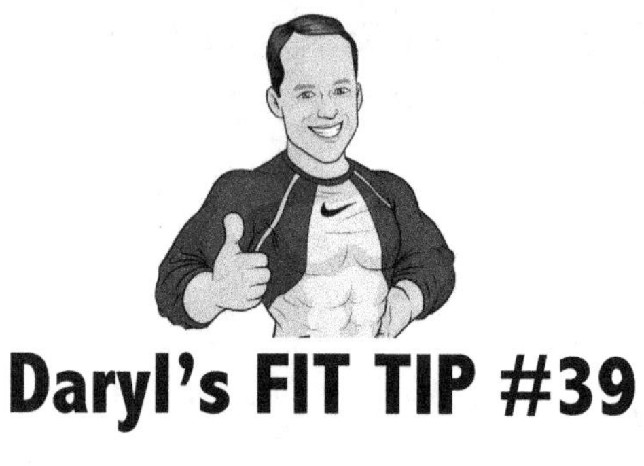

Daryl's FIT TIP #39

NUTRITIONAL PHYSIOLOGY

I don't subscribe to "fad-hype nutrition" programs. I teach nutritional physiology and design meal plans that match a person's physiological makeup.

It boggles my mind how many folks really don't understand how their body works and keep following ridiculous diets or nutritional concepts that are unhealthy. If a person TRULY wants to reduce inflammation, feel better, and reduce body fat they must adhere to a complete overhaul of their nutrition. But unfortunately, too many people are addicted to their junk food or are not willing to make any changes to their lifestyle.

It's rather simple: continue eating and drinking toxins and synthetic compounds-- continue being sick, depressed, anxious, overweight, tired, irritable, angry, low libido, and accelerate aging.

or

Eat wholesome, nutrient-dense, REAL organic food-- and be more productive, more energized, improve body composition, boost immunity, supercharge the brain, put less stress on the liver, pancreas, kidneys and heart, improve sleep, increase libido, and reduce the aging process.

Unfortunately, most people choose the junk food route with a higher risk of disease and accelerated aging, over eating healthy, exercising and reducing the aging effect.

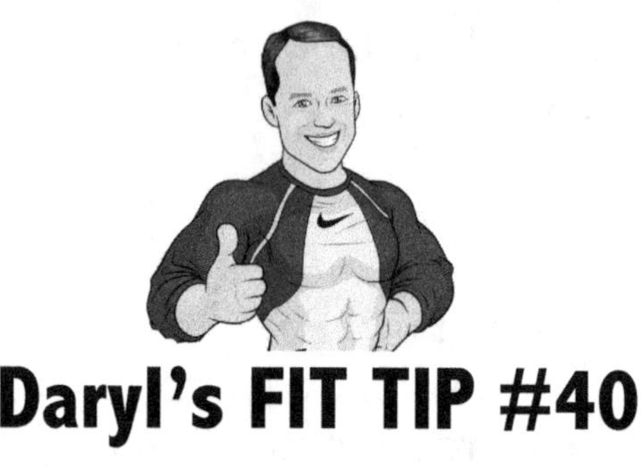

Daryl's FIT TIP #40

STOP and LOOK

We get so busy with our crazy little lives that sometimes we forget to stop and appreciate the magnificent beauty that is all around us. Rather than keeping your head buried in a computer or smartphone, look up and take in nature's POSITOPES to boost your mood and immunity.

Take a deep breath and relax while watching a beautiful sunset. Before you know it all the angst and stress of the day will dissipate.

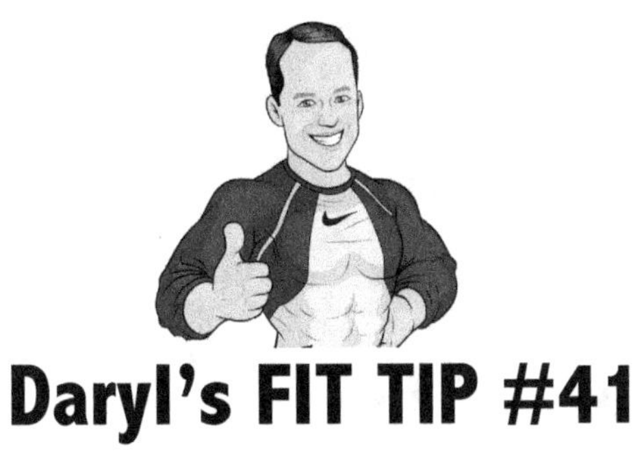

Daryl's FIT TIP #41

VITAL NUTRIENTS

The goal to maintaining a healthy body weight is to feed the active cells with rich vital nutrients. Every organ is like an engine that runs by itself, yet, they work together to keep the whole system alive. Each organ has a specific amount of nutrients to operate efficiently. The only way to supply the necessary amount of vital nutrients is from external food sources.

The BEST food sources are foods loaded with active enzymes.

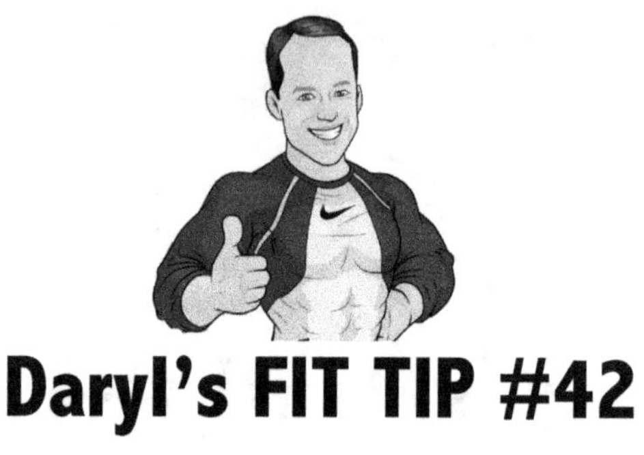

Daryl's FIT TIP #42

NATURALLY

Chemicals don't work, NATURE WORKS! If nature creates a problem, nature creates a solution.

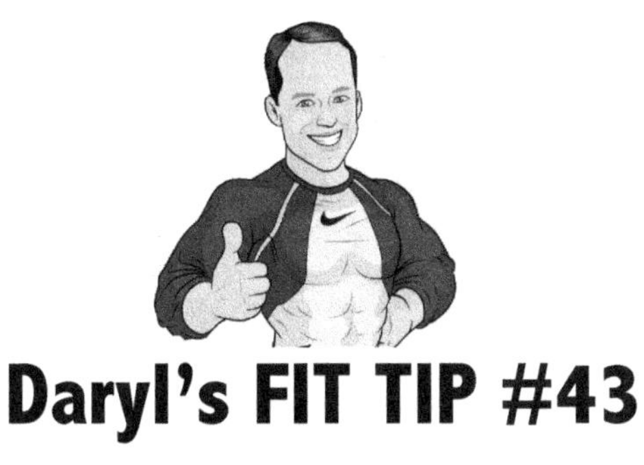

Daryl's FIT TIP #43

HUMAN CONTACT

Human cells are receptors that are stimulated by compounds and energy. Skin cells are very sensitive to the external environment. They become even more active when they come in contact with touch. Skin cells seem to crave contact. Once activated through sensory stimulation in a positive way natural immune-boosting hormones release. Oxytocin, serotonin, dopamine, endorphins, and enkephalins are extremely powerful hormones that when released makes a person feel incredible and super energized. Intimacy is ONE of the best ways to boost your immune system.

So many people develop health problems when they get older. One reason for this is because they no longer have physical human contact. They don't activate the integumentary stimulatory system, losing out on this natural immune boosting phenomenon.

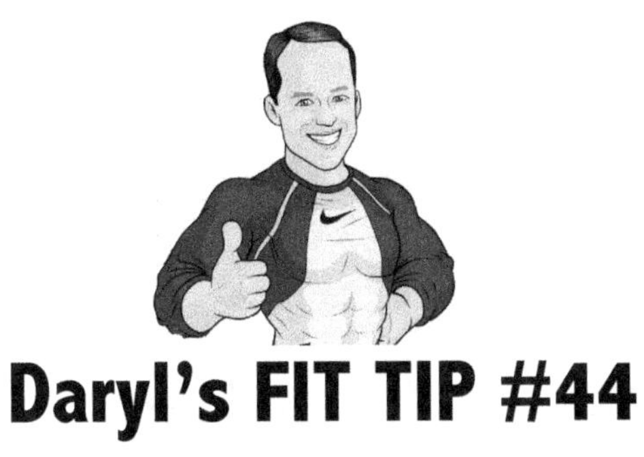

Daryl's FIT TIP #44

SCENT OF HAPPINESS

Your olfactory bulb has a direct connection with the areas of your brain to be crucial in processing emotion and memory, which is why scents can trigger memories in a way a sight or sound doesn't. If you feel yourself feeling glum, take a whiff of whatever reminds you of happier times.

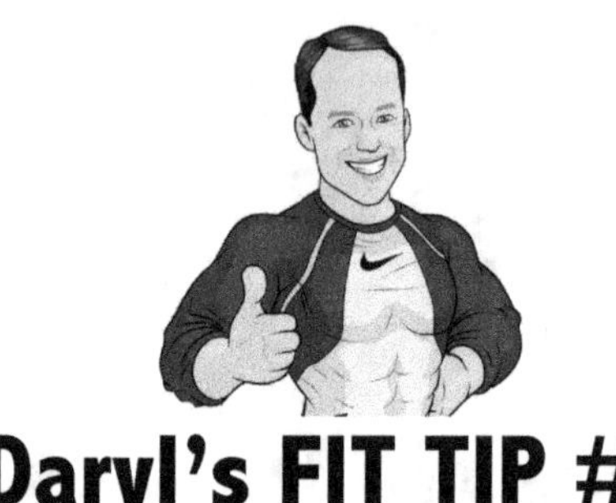

Daryl's FIT TIP #45

NOT A DISEASE

Obesity is NOT a disease. It is a metabolic disorder. 65% of Americans are overweight or OBESE.

The human gene pool is NOT progressing toward a healthier being, it is digressing into a toxic inflamed being. I figured by now in 2018 that humans would be SO much more advanced in health and physical prowess than our ancestors, but the strange thing is our ancestors were healthier. They ate REAL wholesome foods, not this synthetic chemical and sugar ladened garbage that we are subjected to today. No wonder why the physiology of the body is in such disarray affecting many systems of the body, because of the chemicals and junk that is being ingested. I fear that the obesity rate will continue to climb in the years to come and just about everyone will be on some form of medication.

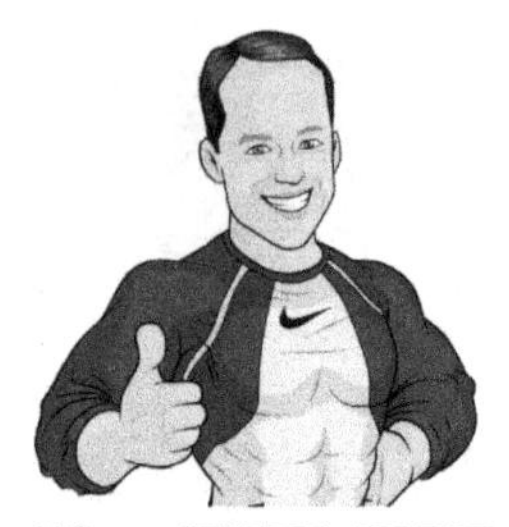

Daryl's FIT TIP #46

BOOSTING NATURAL TESTOSTERONE PRODUCTION

Testosterone is an important anabolic hormone in men and women that help maintain strength, muscle mass, youth, and vitality. This great hormone naturally declines as we age making it harder to maintain: muscle, libido, and youth.

However, boosting the hypothalamic pituitary adrenal gonadal axis (HPAG) by maintaining proper GnRH (Gonadotropin-releasing hormone) secretions from the hypothalamus can help maintain testosterone levels in the body.

GnRH is released by the hypothalamus through rhythmic pulses throughout the day. The morning tends to be the strongest pulse of GnRH production. This would be an ample time to ingest Omega-3 fat. Omega-3 is one of the key components in brain health and GnRH production. The more GnRH produced the greater the HPAG axis is stimulated, ultimately producing more usable testosterone to support muscle mass, youth, and vitality.

This is why I always recommend eating protein and fat first thing upon waking up, to boost the brain and to stimulate the endocrine and reproductive systems.

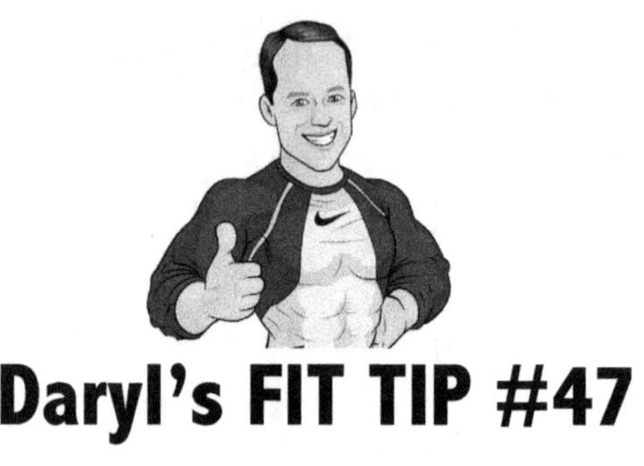

Daryl's FIT TIP #47

CUTTING BACK

Sixty million Americans experience acid reflux at least once a month. Chocolate, coffee, peppermint, tomato products and alcoholic beverages have all been linked to heartburn, and sufferers could see results by simply cutting them out of their diet.

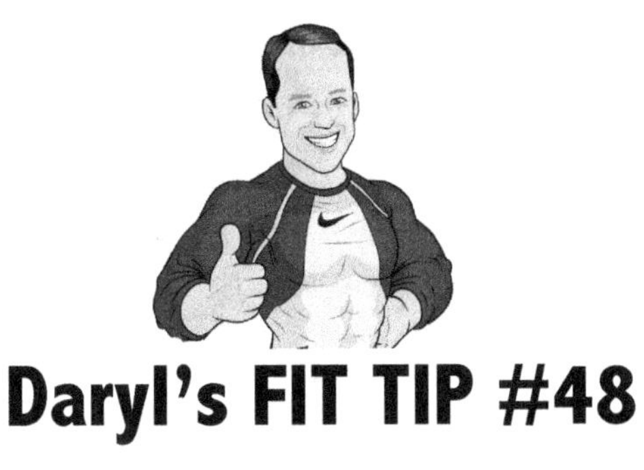

Daryl's FIT TIP #48

FOND MEMORIES

Though we can never physically go back into the past, we can however, think of fond memories from the past. The brain is an incredible computer-like system. It stores endless amounts of data. Whenever the information is restored from our memory banks a neurophysiological shift occurs. Just by thinking of a certain past event the brain will release the hormones associated with that memory as if it was happening in real time.

Whenever you are in a mental funk and can't seem to get out of it, stop and reflect back to a happier time in your life and immerse yourself into that memory. Before you know it you will physiologically feel better. The angst that you were feeling will dissipate. I like to call this effect, the positopic re-shifting effect. You are changing a negative neurological condition into a positive neural condition just by re-thinking your thoughts. It's a great method to use when you are in a stressful situation.

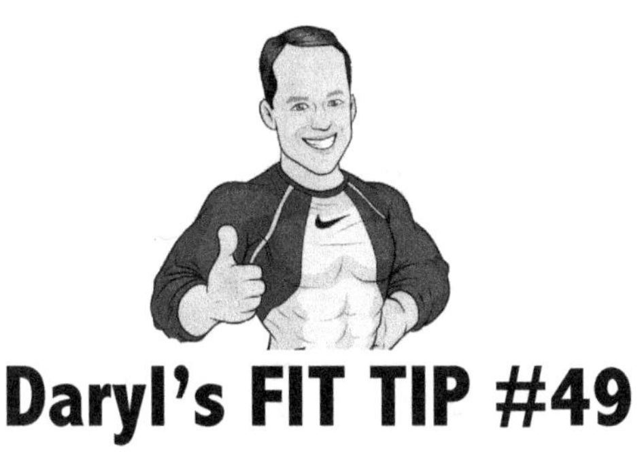

Daryl's FIT TIP #49

BURN MORE FAT

ONE of the BEST ways to burn fat-- WEIGHT TRAIN.

Weight training provides great benefit in building the aerobic and anaerobic enzymes of the muscle. The bigger these enzymes become the more glucose and fat can be metabolized.

During weight training the primary energy source is glucose. And the residual period after weight training the muscle shifts into fat burning. The thermogenic effect (fat burning) can last between 1-8 hours after weight training, depending on the intensities uses.

It takes times to develop the size of the enzymes that is why it is so important to stay on a consistent weight training program. DON'T GIVE UP!!

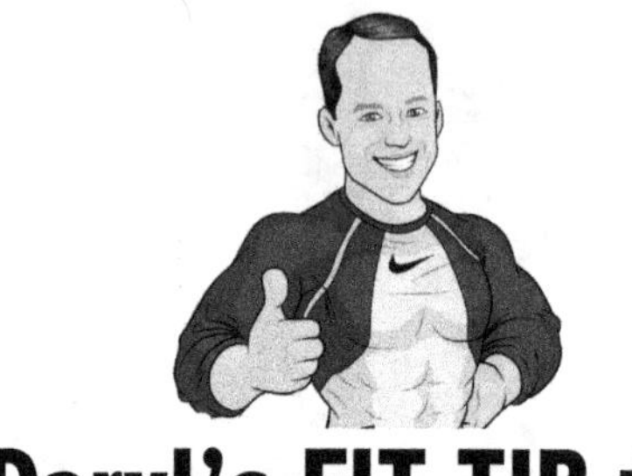

Daryl's FIT TIP #50

FATTY LIVER

If your body looks like the picture below then you suffer from a FATTY LIVER. Drinking alcohol daily (even just one glass per day), eating processed foods, taking medications, and eating sugar contribute to fatty liver. The abdominals protrude, you feel bloated (especially after eating), you belch, sometimes pain in the right shoulder develops, joints ache, and have insomnia, these are all signs of a fatty liver.

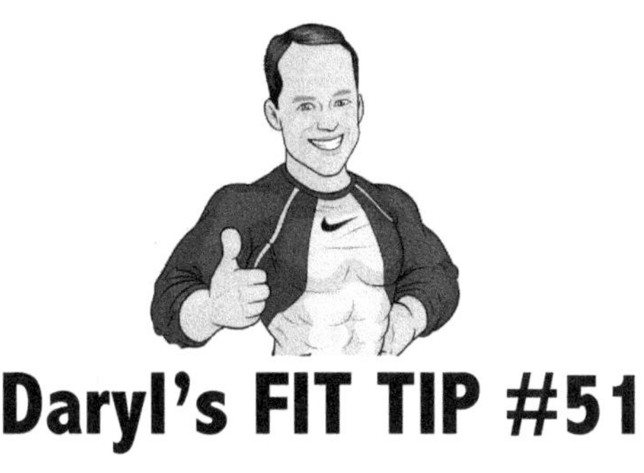

Daryl's FIT TIP #51

AUTOIMMUNE DISEASE

All autoimmune disease is affected by stress. When the body is under stress, whether emotional or physical, the immune system is suppressed. When the immune system is suppressed it cannot defend against destructive pathogens. The pathogens take over and cause problems with the systems of the body. For example, this is why people who suffer from Herpes Simplex (cold sores) have breakouts when they are stressed. This is true of all autoimmune diseases.

The best way to resolve autoimmune flare-ups is to reduce or eliminate stress. It's amazing how the symptoms of an autoimmune flare-up subside once the stressors are reduced or eliminated, the immune system is able to function optimally.

Stress factors include: emotional, physical, chemical, and environmental. Reduce the stress, reduce the reaction.

All autoimmune disease is affected by stress. When the body is under stress, whether emotional or physical, the immune system is suppressed. When the immune system is suppressed it cannot defend against destructive pathogens. The pathogens take over and cause problems with the systems of the body. This is why people who suffer from Herpes Simplex (cold sores) have breakouts when they are stressed. This is true of all autoimmune diseases.

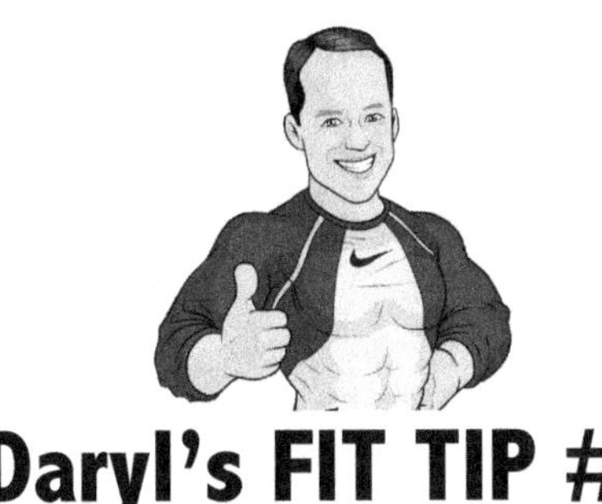

Daryl's FIT TIP #52

BOOST YOUR METABOLISM

Here is a great way to boost your metabolism, exercise in the morning and then again in the evening. You only need 15-20 minutes per session. For some people, this might be an easier option to fit into their busy schedule where training for an hour at a time is not realistic.

Exercising in small increments throughout the day can increase your active metabolism, which can help burn extra sugar and fat. And it helps to increase dopamine, serotonin, and noradrenaline levels. You do not need to go crazy, just taking a brisk walk in the morning and then again in the evening can do wonders. Even better, lifting weights in the evening can really boost your metabolism.

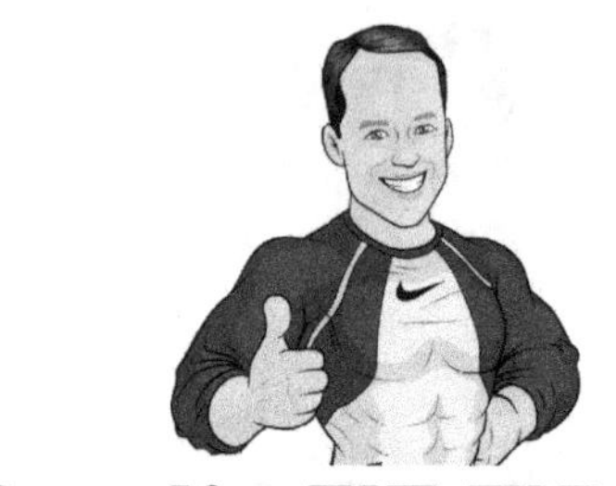

Daryl's FIT TIP #53

GOUT

Gout is a common and complex form of arthritis that can affect anyone. It's characterized by sudden, severe attacks of pain, swelling, redness and tenderness in the joints, often the joint at the base of the big toe.

Here are my recommendations for helping resolve gout symptoms:

1. Celery Seed Extract (Supplement form is fine). Helps reduce Uric Acid. Or eat celery sticks throughout the day, plain with nothing on it.
2. Black Cherry Juice Extract. Buy in concentrated form, dilute in water.
3. Cod Liver Oil (Supplement) take in evening before bedtime.
4. Magnesium (Supplement)
5. Potassium Citrate (Supplement

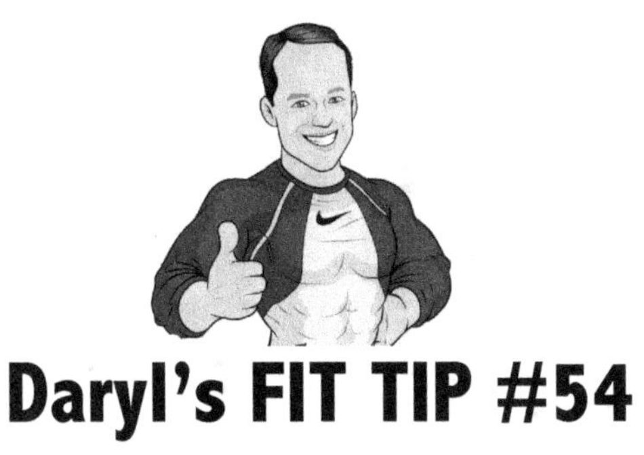

Daryl's FIT TIP #54

POSITIVITY

When you process negitopes you produce negative molecules in your body resulting in negative energy. Negative energy manifests into disease.

Attracting yourself to positopes will produce positive molecules in your body resulting in a boost in positive energy, which will improve the health and functions of all the systems of the body.

My book Positopes™ provides strategies on how to reduce the toxic inflammation of the body. It can be purchased on Amazon, Barnes and Noble, and my own website. www.darylconant.com

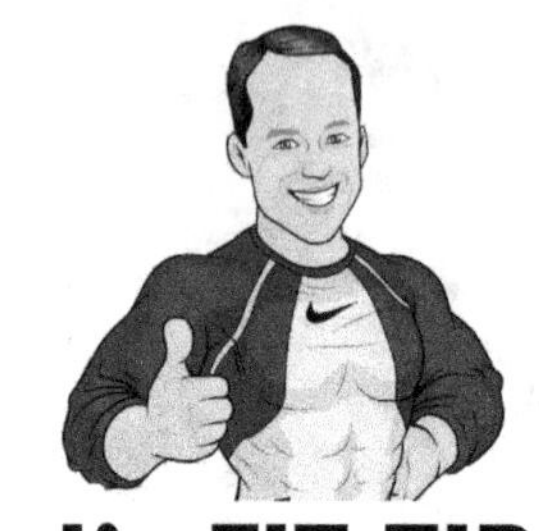

Daryl's FIT TIP #55

WHAT I EAT

I am often asked, "Daryl what do you eat for breakfast?" And my answer is, "I eat healthy fat and protein, NO SUGAR! Eating sugar first thing in the morning will put your metabolism into a tailspin, which will cause energy depletion and sugar cravings throughout the day.

The best is to eat only fat, protein, and veggies for breakfast. I will make an omelet with spinach and mushrooms. There is enough fat in the eggs to sustain my energy for hours.

The WORST breakfast is: A glass of Orange juice (90% Sugar), a bowl of processed high carb cereal (90% sugar), a banana (Sugar), and White Toast (Sugar) with Jam (100% Sugar). This combination will promote many metabolic problems and will cause an energy crash within 2 hours. Once this occurs the body craves more sugar.

Remember this: When sugar is the main fuel fat cannot be burned. Fat can only be burned off through fat metabolism. Sugar chain eating (eating sugar every 3-4 hours) will cause weight gain inhibiting fat burning.

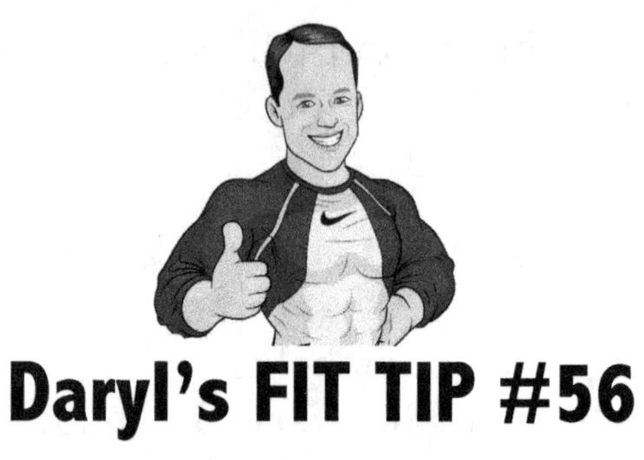

Daryl's FIT TIP #56

WHAT'S COOKING?

For more awesome meal ideas check out my cookbook, it's loaded with D-lisciousness ☺ :) You can order it right off my website www.darylconant.com

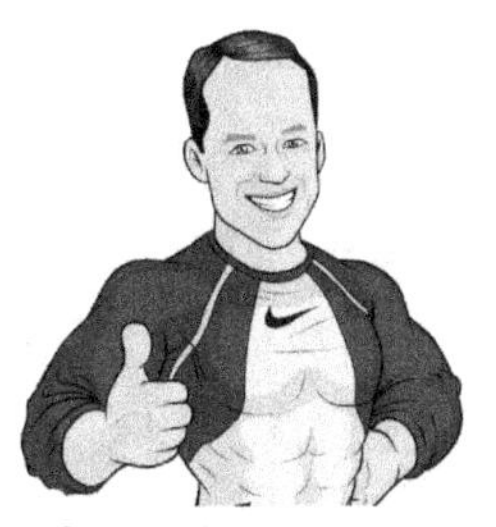

Daryl's FIT TIP #57

GOOD NEWS CHOCOLATE LOVERS

Here is a GREAT little snack to boost a high level of antioxidants into your body- DARK CHOCOLATE and BLUEBERRIES. A 1/2 ounce of 85% or higher organic dark chocolate with a small handful of organic blueberries is my recommended serving size. DON'T go crazy, you only need a little to get the benefits.

85% or higher organic dark chocolate has proven to be loaded with organic compounds that are biologically active and function as antioxidants. These include polyphenols, flavanols, and catechins, among others. The flavanols in dark chocolate can stimulate the endothelium, the lining of arteries, to produce nitric oxide.The flavonols can protect against sun damage, improve blood flow to the skin and increase skin density and hydration.

Dark chocolate can also reduce insulin resistance, which is another common risk factor for many diseases like heart disease and diabetes. And it also contains theobromine, which may be a key reason why it can improve brain function.

Blueberries are ranked number ONE in antioxidants. They contain a high level of Vitamin C, anthocyanin, the selenium, the vitamins A, B-complex, and E, zinc, sodium, potassium, copper, magnesium, phosphorus, manganese etc, in addition, blueberries may help reduce belly fat, improve vision, and risk factors for cardiovascular disease and metabolic syndrome. Blueberries help keep the urinary tract preventing infections and can prevent and heal neurotic disorders by preventing degeneration and death of neurons, brain-cells and also by restoring the health of the central nervous system.

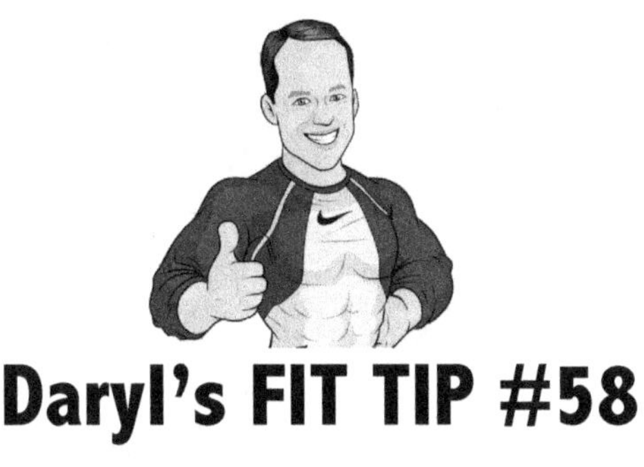

Daryl's FIT TIP #58

PROPER NUTRITION

Every BODY has a specific metabolic demand. This is based on genetic factors as well as physiological factors. However, no matter if you are a slow, medium, or fast oxidizer it is important to always take in the proper amount of usable nutrients to feed the systems of the body. Each system has a specific nutrient demand, which must be replenished on a daily basis. Unfortunately, many people are NUTRIENT DEPRIVED and suffer from body composition imbalance.

Being nutrient deprived will cause a plethora of health problems, both emotionally and physically. In order to maintain physiological stability, it is IMPERATIVE that you follow the laws of nature and adhere to a COMPLETE BALANCE of nutrients.

One of BIGGEST mistakes is cutting nutrient intake down below your resting metabolic rate, this is a dangerous thing to do. The theory of eating less and exercise is misleading to many people. To lose body fat it is important to eat a little less than what you expend but not to go below your resting metabolic nutrient demand. Starving the systems of their required nutrients will cause negative feedback loops forcing a person into catabolic chaos. Being in catabolism for long periods of time can actually damage the endocrine system.

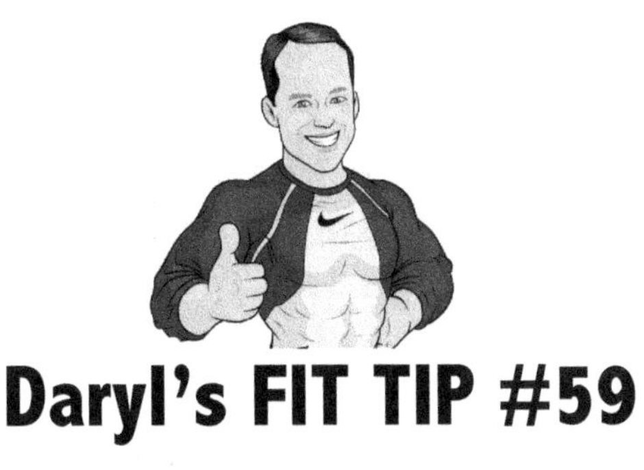

Daryl's FIT TIP #59

WHY CAN THEY?

Have you ever wondered why some people can eat anything they want and NEVER gain any weight? This is because of the weight-regulating mechanisms built within their physiological systems of the body to allow efficient fat and sugar metabolism. Here are a few of those factors:

1. Fast Resting Metabolic Rate: Having a fast resting metabolic rate allows a person to consume more food to keep up with the metabolic demand.

2. More Brown Fat: Naturally lean folks tend to have more brown fat. Brown fat is different from the "storage" fat in that it has the ability to burn part of the food you eat and waste the excess energy as heat so it doesn't have to be stored as fat.

3.   Efficient   Cellular   Sodium-Potassium Pumps: Sodium and potassium is pumped repeatedly across the cell membranes of billions of cells in the body. This pump uses energy and is driven by an enzyme called sodium-potassium ATP-ase. Thin people have much higher levels of sodium-potassium ATP-ase than the obese and can therefore waste excess energy much more easily.

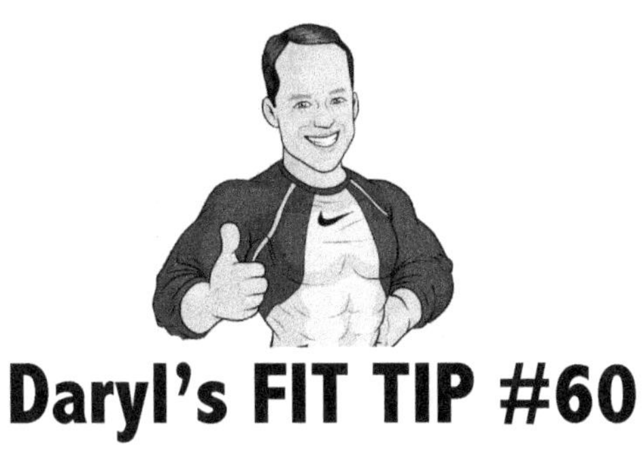

Daryl's FIT TIP #60

EXERCISE ADDICTION

There is no doubt that exercise is one of the best things you can do for your health, however, overtraining can be dangerous to your health.

The endorphin rush from exercise produces a sense of euphoria. It is easy for a person to get addicted to the endorphin rush, especially when a person is dealing with emotional or physical conflict. The endorphin rush helps numb the pain. But exercising too much will actually dampen the endorphin rush making it less effective over time, which will cause the person to keep exercising to try and get their fix of endorphin release. Unfortunately, too much exercise will cause an excess of tissue breakdown causing the immune system to weaken. This will put a person into a catabolic shift that will inhibit proper protein synthesis and restoration of the physiological systems leading to health problems.

Here is a list of symptoms from overtraining:
* Muscle wasting,
* Fat gain,
* Joint pain
* Diarrhea,
* Depression,
* Anxiety,
* Severe weight loss,
* Menstrual problems
* Hair loss,
* Loss of appetite,
* Irritability
* Emotional firestorms (crying, moody, melancholy
* Anger
* Low libido
* Insomnia
* Emaciated features
* Poor muscle tone
* Sugar cravings
* Ketoacidosis
* Rhabdomyolysis
* Blood in urine
* Lackluster

* Short fused temper
* Poor performance
* Weakness in legs, arms
* Migraines
* Nausea

Avoid overtraining at all costs.

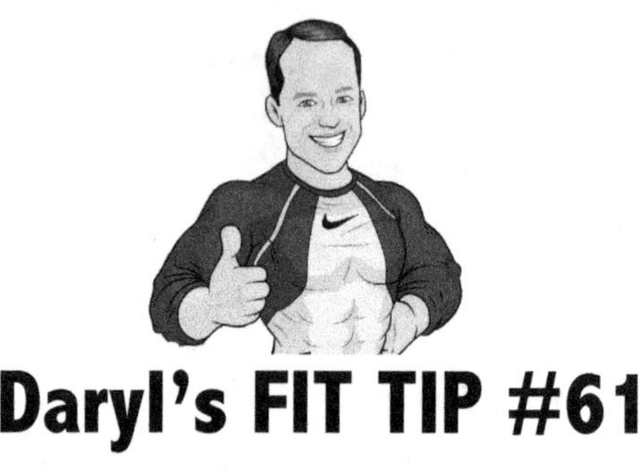

Daryl's FIT TIP #61

APPROVED FRUIT

In general, fruits are quite nutrient dense. Eating too much fruit during the day can cause blood sugar levels to get too high, which could cause fat gain as a result of insulin pushing the sugar out of the bloodstream and into fat cells if the muscles or liver can't absorb it.

There are many fruits that I consider high glycemic and should be eaten sparingly (i.e., melons, bananas. However, there are some fruits that I consider worthy of eating purely for their anti-oxidant and anti-inflammation properties: blueberries, goji berries, pomegranate, strawberries, Acai berries, cranberries, Acerola cherries, grapes, black cherries.

These fruits have incredible nutrient value and are POWERFULL IMMUNITY BOOSTERS. I suggest eating these types of fruits in small amounts on days that you are exercising. This is because if you happen to over-consume them the extra sugar will most likely get absorbed by the muscles or liver due to glycogen depletion rather than going into fat cells.

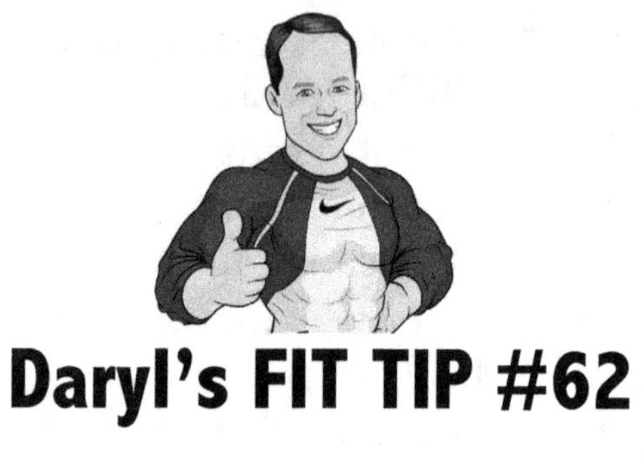

Daryl's FIT TIP #62

NOTHING BEATS

Nothing beats eating REAL NUTRIENT DENSE ORGANIC NATURAL food for keeping the body healthy.

My motto is: If the food entering your mouth isn't from a source of food that could be obtained 100 years ago then don't consume it. Natural food is the ONLY way, man-made food stay away.

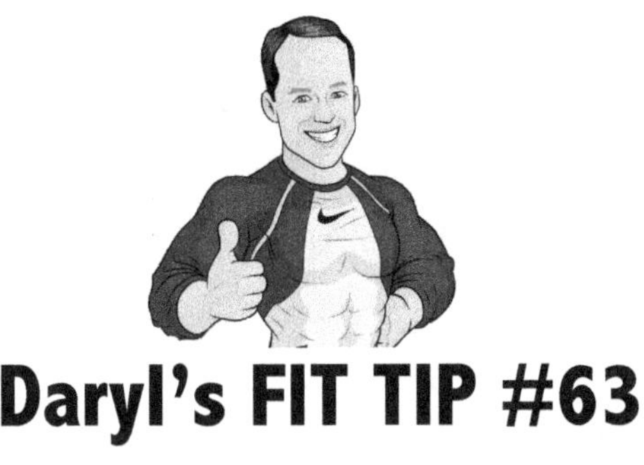

Daryl's FIT TIP #63

UNDERSTANDING ENERGY BALANCE

There is one basic truth to fat loss. You need to burn more than you eat. Having your RESTING METABOLIC RATE tested can help determine how fast your metabolism is and how many calories your body burn daily. Then you can calculate precisely how much food you need per day to maintain your energy requirement. Knowing this will solve the weight gain problem because you won't be consuming more than what your body needs. I made up the chart below to illustrate energy output and energy input. (The calorie expenditure numbers are from a previous test, used as an example for my illustration).

Maintenance Zone:

Once you reach your goal weight, this is how many calories your body needs to maintain your weight.

Fat Loss Zone:
Healthy fat loss comes from eating slightly less than your body needs. By eating healthy foods throughout the day you should not feel hungry.

Medically Supervised Zone:
Very low nutrient diets should only be done under medical supervision. Supervision is required to ensure adequate nutrition and to monitor and treat the potential showing of metabolic rate.

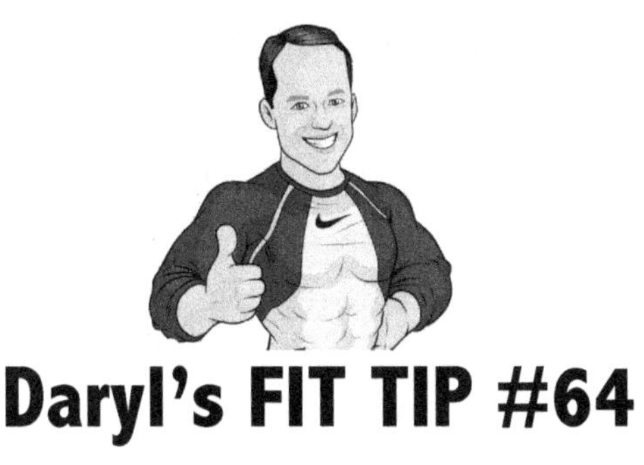

Daryl's FIT TIP #64

REST DAY

One of the most overlooked components of training is taking time off to rest. Many people will exercise every day because they feel that if they take a day off that they might put on body fat, or lose their gains. This will not happen.

Exercise breaks down tissue and depletes the cells. Many days without rest will actually weaken the physiological integrity of the body systems, which will increase risk of injury and mental acuity. The only time the body restores rebuilds and replenishes is through REST. It can take 24-72 hours for the cellular machinery to fully get restored after an exercise bout. The nervous system needs 72 hours to fully recharge the nerves. Muscle needs 48 hours to fully recover. The cardiovascular system only needs 24 hours to fully recover.

YOU NEVER GROW or BUILD THE CELLS during exercise, you break them down. Exercise is a forced catabolic event. During REST and SLEEP is when you REBUILD the body, making it stronger, healthier and more enduring.

I recommend taking at least 1-2 days off a week every week. And taking 4-5 days off in a row after every 6 weeks of training.

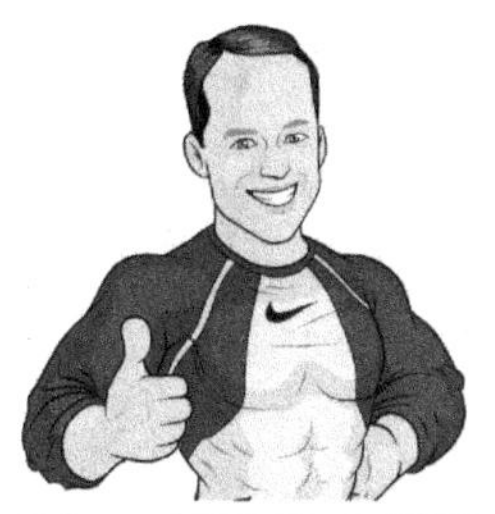

Daryl's FIT TIP #65

IT'S ABOUT THYME, for crying out loud...

The herb thyme is a powerful evergreen shrub has many health benefits.

* Anti-fungal Properties. Thyme contains thymol, which can help against fungal and viral infections.

* Anti-oxidant Power. The phenolic antioxidants found in thyme, including lutein, zeaxanthin, and thymonin contribute to neutralizing and eliminating free radicals throughout the body. These antioxidants help prevent oxidative stress present in your organs, as well as your neural pathways, heart, eyes, and skin.

* Better Circulation. Iron and other minerals found in thyme can help stimulate red blood cells, which increases oxygen capacity in the body.

* Heart Health. The potassium and manganese in thyme helps keep the cardiovascular regulated reducing the build up of plaque (Atherosclerosis)

* Boosts Immunity. Thyme has Vitamin C, which is one of the most powerful immune vitamins in the body. Vitamin C stimulates the production of white blood cells, which are the first line of defense in the body's immune system. Vitamin C also plays a crucial part in the production of collagen, which is essential for the creation and repair of cells, muscles, tissues, and blood vessels.

* Stress Reduction. Thyme has vitamin B-6 a powerful mood stabilizer. Vitamin B-6 helps regulate neurotransmitters providing a calming effect.

* Respiratory Relief. Thyme helps defend against respiratory illnesses and bronchitis, chronic asthma, congestion, colds, flu, blocked sinuses or seasonal allergies, thyme acts as an expectorant and an anti-inflammatory substance.

I recommend just dicing up some raw thyme and putting it on your salad. You don't need a lot, just 2-3 diced tablespoons sprinkled on top of your salad is all you need to get these great benefits.

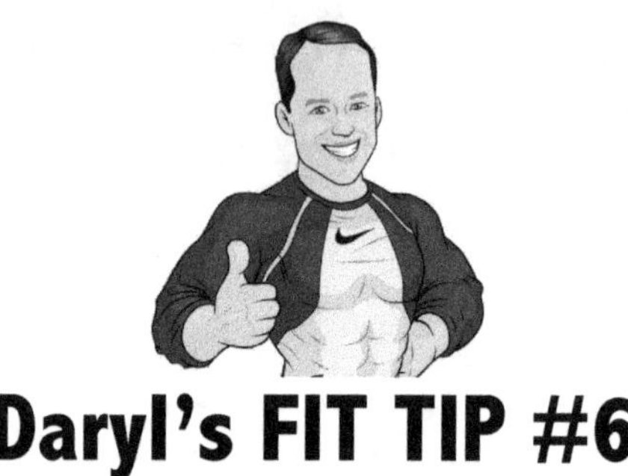

Daryl's FIT TIP #66

STAY HYDRATED

One of the single most important and easiest things you can do for your body is to drink enough water. Here are my 8 steps for keeping optimally hydrated.

1. Drink half your body weight in ounces of water a day.

2. Drink early. Don't wait for thirst to hit. By the time you feel the urge to hoist a glass, you're already on your way to dehydration.

3. Sip slow and steady. Don't gulp all the day's water at once, the overload will just have you rushing to the restroom.

4. Adjust as necessary. If you are working out, tack on another 15 to 20 ounces per hour of exertion.

5. Beat the heat. If the temperature is rising, add another 8 ounces per hour outside. Add 20 or more ounces per hour if you are exercising in the heat.

6. Sub in sources. Having trouble drinking water? Add in vegetables. Vegetables retain water and when you consume them you will also extract the water from the vegetable.

7. Spice up your routine. Add some kick to the hydration process to keep it interesting. A slice of lemon, lime or cucumber can add a new flavor to boost a plain ole glass of H2O.

8. Schedule in a time to drink. Older brains may not sense dehydration and lose the ability to send out the signals for thirst. Set times to drink and stick to them.

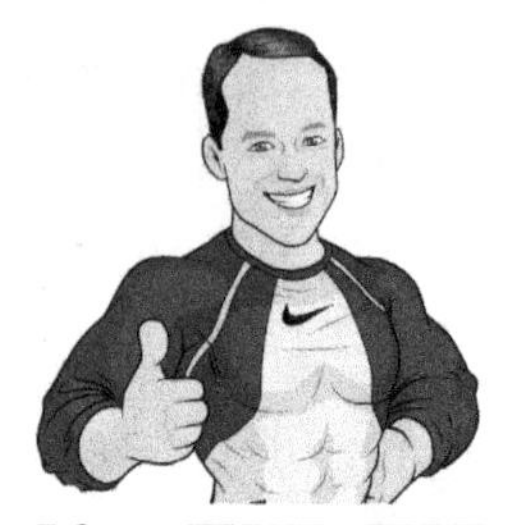

Daryl's FIT TIP #67

HOW TO AVOID WRINKLES

Call them character or laugh lines if you want, but they are still just wrinkles going incognito. Time is going to give everyone a few lines on their face. But how deep-set, and noticeable, the face furrows are reflect, in large part, how good a caretaker of your skin--and your entire--body you are. Since skin is your body's largest organ, fending off worsening wrinkles is mostly about adopting an overall healthy lifestyle. Here are my recommendations for cutting encroaching creases off at the pass.

1. Eat healthy. Nutrient dense foods that contain vitamins A,B,C, E, and good fats all help keep skin healthy.

2. Get a little help. Supplements can help keep a high level of skin smoothing

compounds in your body to help promote healthy skin. Omega 3s, krill oil, and evening primrose oil; alpha-lipoic acid; hyraluronic acid are essential for maintaining healthy skin.

3. Drink up. Dehydration plays a big role in the formation of wrinkles. Water also helps clear out toxins that are built up in the skin.

4. Stop smoking PERIOD!!!

5. Move more. Exercise helps improve blood and oxygen flow throughout the entire body. Also, sweating cleans the skin by removing toxins.

6. Moisturize. Using Moisturizer on your skin draws more water into skin cells, preventing wrinkles.

7. Slough off the old. Getting rid of dead skin cells by exfoliating may not stop wrinkles altogether, but it will go a long way toward making the ones you have less noticeable.

8. Factor in the sun. Ninety percent of wrinkles treated by dermatologists are caused by excessive sun exposure. Limit sun exposure to a minimum throughout the day. No more than 10-15 of sun exposure.

9. Get your beauty sleep. Catching an adequate amount of ZZZ's is key in staving off wrinkles, because of a hormone called HGH (human growth hormone). This hormone makes cells grow and reproduce, keeping skin healthy.

10 Don't OVERDO THE JOE. Caffeine restricts blood vessels, making it harder to supply the skin with nutrients.

11. RELAX. People who are stressed out all the time seem to wrinkle up faster than folks who are calm and relaxed. This is because a person under stress is activating the sympathetic nervous system, which constricts cells. The face expressions will tend to be angry or furrowed causing deep embedded wrinkles. You can tell a lot about a person with the type and number of wrinkles on their face.

12. STOP washing your face excessively. Using a facecloth and scrubbing hard around your eyes and face will cause wrinkles. The cells around the eyes are very sensitive and fragile, when you scrub this area you remove thousands of cells exposing the area to damage. It is necessary to preserve the natural oils of the skin around the eyes to

keep the area healthy. Just apply light pressure and gently wash the area with your hands and not a facecloth.

13. Limit alcohol. Alcohol is a toxic compound that dehydrates water in the body, which means less water and nutrients for the skin.

14. Eliminate processed sugar. Processed sugar causes inflammation in the body. The skin is directly affected by the inflammation. Poor skin health is directed linked to the damaging effects of processed sugar, which increasing accelerated aging and wrinkles.

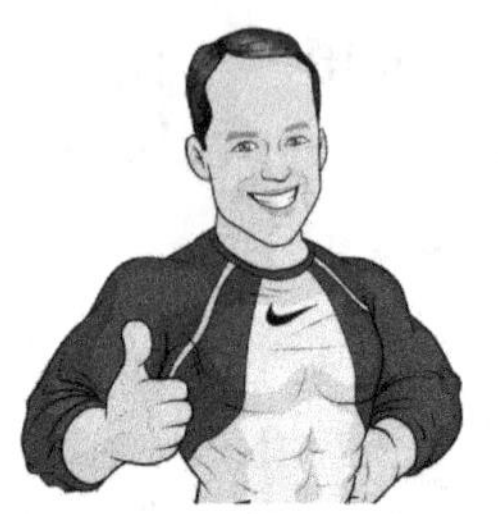

Daryl's FIT TIP #68

HONEY, Natures Natural Sweetener

A power food that is often neglected is REAL NATURAL HONEY. During an intense workout your muscles lose glycogen (muscle sugar). It is important to restore glycogen levels quickly after exercise to avoid staying in catabolism (breakdown), which could result in muscle wasting. Having a tablespoon of REAL NATURAL HONEY immediately after a workout will restore glycogen levels.

It has to be the REAL kind of honey straight from the hive-- raw and not processed in any way. REAL NATURAL HONEY looks like a paste rather than a liquid. The liquid form of honey has been processed and the natural enzymes have been destroyed due to the heating process.

REAL NATURAL HONEY is loaded with vitamins and minerals and enough glucose to replenish depleted muscle tissue.

Honey can also be used as a natural sweetener to give certain foods a little sweetness.

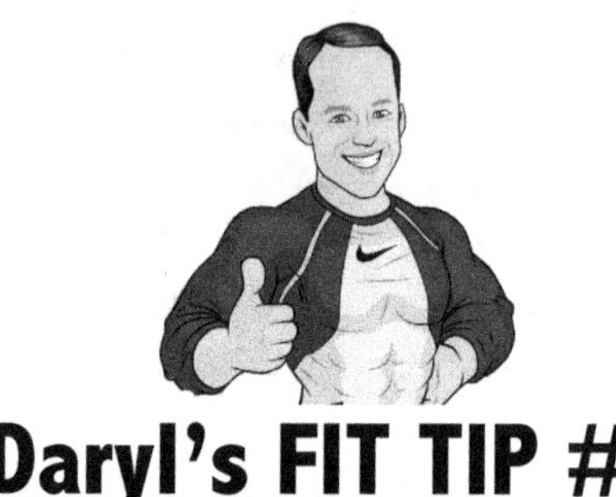

Daryl's FIT TIP #69

VALUES

What makes a person who they are, is built upon their values as a human being. A person's character is based on their own values. What we learn and how we interpret from right and wrong is the foundation of our stream of consciousness. We become plasteurized into a certain belief system that becomes us. This belief system defines who we are. This projection of our self is viewed by others and is processed through the higher channels of consciousness to represent a certain identity. Depending on the values that have been instilled within the stream of consciousness will decide how the identity of a person is perceived. Everyone has certain values that they have formed to project against the various frequencies and channels within the mass of collective energy. Values get transferred into the energy flow of the body. The body has two forms of energy; negative and positive. Negative energy decreases the efficiency of the physiological systems, whereas positive energy boosts the efficiency of the physiological systems. Depending on the values formed will decide how a person handles adversity. We can decide to become a monster reverting to unconscious primal tendencies to stir up conflict, or we can decide to become a higher form of intelligence and consciousness to defeat conflict.

Through your belief system and stored values determines the type of energy you become; negative or positive. Negative energy destroys happiness and creates conflict. Positive energy solidifies happiness and overrides conflict.

Everything we project from our stream of consciousness is based on our own values.

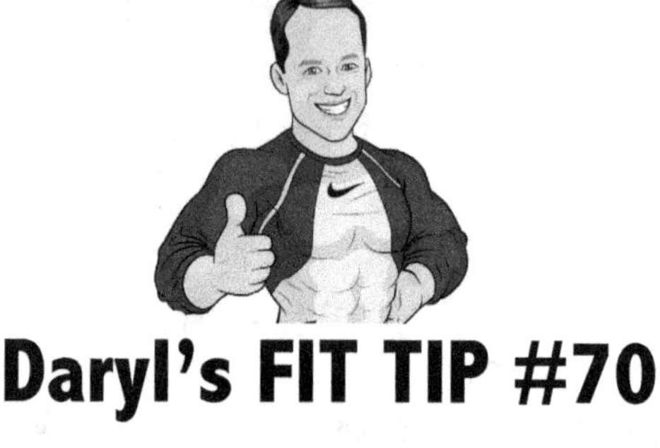

Daryl's FIT TIP #70

HOW YOU THINK CAN MAKE YOU FAT

You don't even have to eat and you can put on FAT. The brain is the control center of the body and connected to a vast network of nerves that transmit signals throughout every part of the body. Everything that we process in the brain sets off synapses. These synapses are transferred into either electrical or chemical output. The synapse travels down the axon and ends up causing an action potential. At the axon terminal, a certain neurotransmitter is released causing a certain reaction to the target cell. This incredible sequence occurs every second of life.

Being anxious, worried, fearful, angry, depressed, embarrassed, uptight, frustrated, annoyed, hateful, are all emotions that stimulate the amygdala in the brain. The amygdala sends signals to the HPA axis (hypothalamus, pituitary, adrenal). The HPA axis is connected to the sympathetic nervous system. The SNS is the "fight of flight" control system. When the SNS is turned on it uses sugar as it's main fuel source. Blood sugar and stored sugar gets used up really fast during a SNS response. When there is a surge of sugar in the blood, insulin is released to regulate blood sugar. Insulin causes the cells to open up to clear the sugar. One place that sugar goes is fat cells. Another problem is that fat metabolism ceases during insulin secretion and growth hormone levels also drop.

This entire sequence can occur all day long just from the way you think. Now, once the sugar is depleted from the SNS response, your brain begins to crave sugar because your brain's primary fuel is sugar. So you go and start consuming high sugary foods. Again, high levels of sugar enters the bloodstream and insulin is secreted to regulate the high blood sugar. Thus, the entire SNS sequence is activated. If you don't consume sugar and deprive yourself of food, your liver will convert your OWN MUSCLE tissue into glucose to be used to fuel the SNS. This will also cause fat to remain in storage.

Remember this: YOU CANNOT BURN FAT DURING a SNS response. YOU CANNOT BURN FAT in the presence of INSULIN. YOU CANNOT BURN FAT when sugar is the primary fuel source. How you think can directly affect your nervous system activating the sympathetic nervous system all day long.

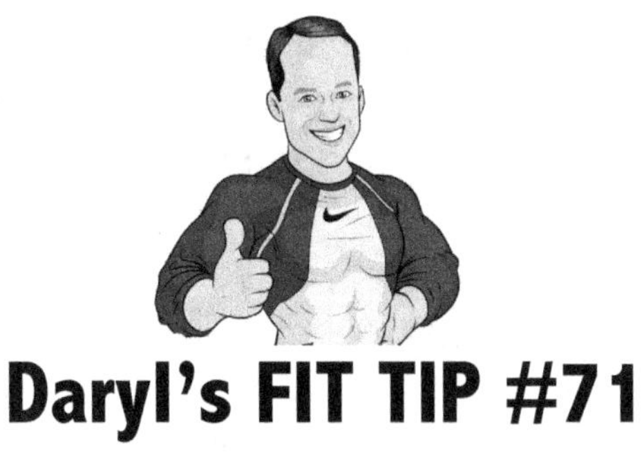

Daryl's FIT TIP #71

LOW BACK/HAMSTRING ISSUES?
Run Backwards.

If you do quad dominant exercises, running, cycling, squatting, or sit all day, and suffer from lower back pain, hamstring tightness/pain you could be suffering from musculoskeletal imbalance. Here is a way to improve musculoskeletal imbalance-- run backward

When I suggest running backward to my clients they all look at me like I have lost my mind, but it actually works. Performing quad dominant exercises over time will cause muscle imbalance. The quads get too developed putting too much tension on the lower back and hamstring forcing them to be overly tight. Hamstring pulls and herniated discs are common problems.

Running backward will activate the extensors of the posterior kinetic chain taking the stress off the quadriceps. The hamstrings and glutes will become the prime movers. Challenging the neuromuscular system in this unorthodox pattern will strengthen the contractibility factors of the hamstrings and glutes, which will help correct musculoskeletal imbalance.

If you don't want to run on the road backward, then I suggest you do Retro Treadmill. Put the elevation of the treadmill to 7-degree incline and walk backward, do not run. Keep the speed between 3-4 mph. Go for a distance of 1-3 miles, your glutes and hamstrings will be burning.

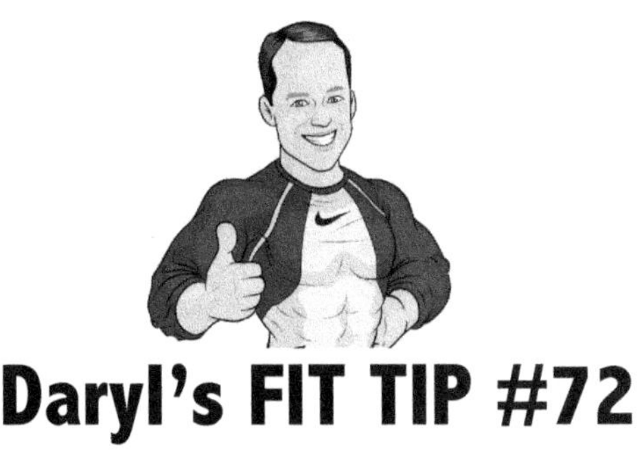

Daryl's FIT TIP #72

NUTRIENT NEEDS

The more you exercise, the more tissue you break down, therefore the more nutrients you have to consume to repair and rebuild the tissue. IT MAKES NO SENSE to eat less nutrients than your body needs to support lean body mass, this only increases the CATABOLIC effect, which will ultimately cause muscle wasting.

People who train a lot and don't eat enough nutrients tend to develop more subcutaneous fat and cellulite because of the muscle wasting. The smoothness of their muscles is dimpled with fat. To try and remedy the situation they EXERCISE even more and continue to eat less nutrients. It's a never-ending cycle.

Remember: The MORE YOU EXERCISE the MORE NUTRIENTS you need to eat.

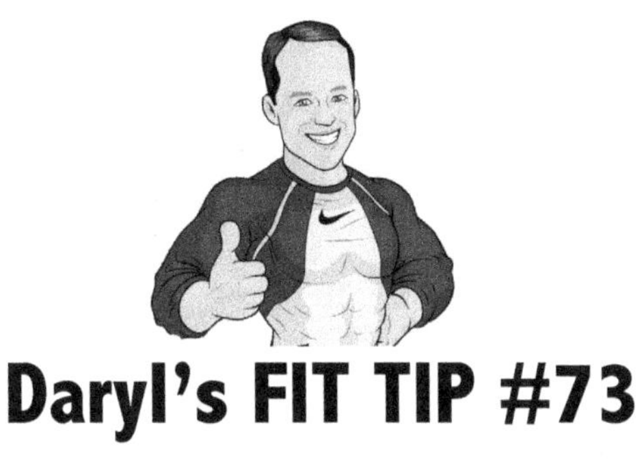

Daryl's FIT TIP #73

YOUR MOM WAS RIGHT

Like mom always said, "eat your vegetables." Moms know best. When I was a young lad and started getting serious about bodybuilding I knew that I needed to eat vegetables to get the nutrients my body needed, but I didn't like vegetables. When there were vegetables on my plate I would hide them in my napkin and pretended that I ate them. Then I realized in order to build muscle I needed more vegetables so I would hold my nose and eat them really fast to try an avoid the taste.

Over the years I have gotten to really love the taste of vegetables. I eat 7-10 different types of vegetables every day. It is important to consume 7-10 cups of vegetables every day to get the nutrient benefit. One of the key minerals for the body is potassium. The body needs 4700 mg. of potassium a day. Most people don't even come close to taking in their recommended daily allowance of potassium. Some people think if they eat a banana that they are getting enough potassium-- WRONG! It would take about 14 bananas to get 4700 mg of potassium.

I recommend my SUPER SALAD and it is one of the awesome dishes I have listed in my FIT COOKBOOK. All the veggies are raw and loaded with nutrients. The taste is INCREDIBLE! My mouth is watering just writing this tip. There are over 10 vegetables in this salad. I will have a protein along with it. This lunch will provide me energy for hours. It is D-liscious!!

FOLKS you don't need gimmick drinks, or potions, or pills, or hype. You just need to eat REAL FOOD.

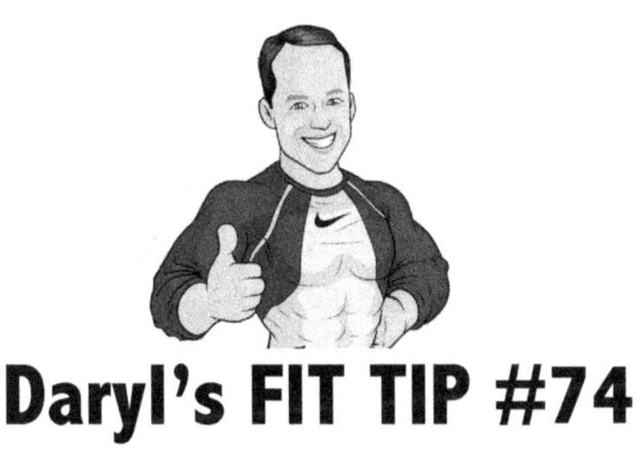

Daryl's FIT TIP #74

THERMOGENIC BOOST

To accelerate fat burning it is essential to increase the activate metabolic rate of the muscles. When the muscles are worked and heated up the residual thermogenic effect (fat burning) can last from 2-8 hours depending on the type of exercise and intensity.

Here is a great way to boost your thermogenesis into higher gear. Exercise for 15-20 minutes in the morning and then again in the evening for 15-20 minutes at high intensity. For example, you could weight train in the morning and then do wind sprints in the evening. Splitting up the exercise will provide an increase in fat burning because of the long-lasting thermogenic effect. Exercising at a high intensity for long periods is not advantageous. The more volume and intensity in less time equals greater power output of the muscles. The muscles cannot sustain high-intensity for a long duration.

You can only perform a high-intensity exercise for a short duration because natural HGH (human growth hormone) levels drop quickly. When HGH levels get low, cortisol levels increase. Cortisol will dampen the anabolic effect.

The key is to activate as much muscle as possible to burn as much fat as possible. In order to burn fat, the MUSCLE TISSUE MUST BE HEATED UP. You don't burn fat when you are exercising at high intensities, you burn stored glycogen (sugar). You burn fat during the recovery phase following the exercise session as the body is restoring homeostasis. The more intense the exercise the longer the residual thermogenic effect lasts.

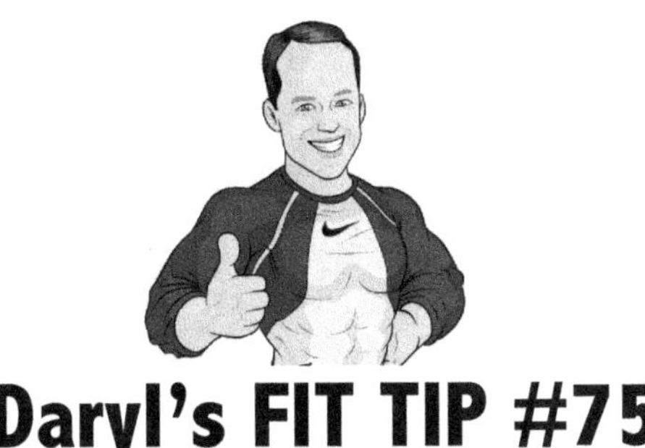

Daryl's FIT TIP #75

LOST MUSCLE PUMP

You are training and suddenly the muscles lose tone, blood volume and feel cold and soft. No matter how much you try to continue to stimulate the muscle it won't get "pumped" again during that session. The muscle actually shrinks right before your eyes. The reason for this is because the muscle has been overstimulated and cortisol has been released inhibiting the Beta-2 adrenergic receptors. Beta-2 adrenergic receptors are responsible for glycogenolysis (breakdown of glucose) within muscle tissue. Since the muscle is depleted cortisol attaches to the receptors to turn off anaerobic metabolism. Blood is then diverted away from the target muscle to protect from further cellular damage.

In order to get the muscles to feel full and powerful again, they must go through the restoration cycle. Going from a sympathetic nervous system response (exercise) increases the need for cellular repair. During rest, especially sleep, the cellular machinery of the muscles get repaired and restored. Glycogen levels (sugar) can only get replenished and protein synthesis is most active when the body is in the parasympathetic nervous system mode.

In order to refill depleted glycogen levels, it is important to consume carbohydrates during the resting phase. Not junk carbohydrates, but healthy carbohydrates like fruit and vegetables. Once you restore the glycogen levels and protein synthesis rebuilds the cellular machinery your muscles will feel full and powerful again.

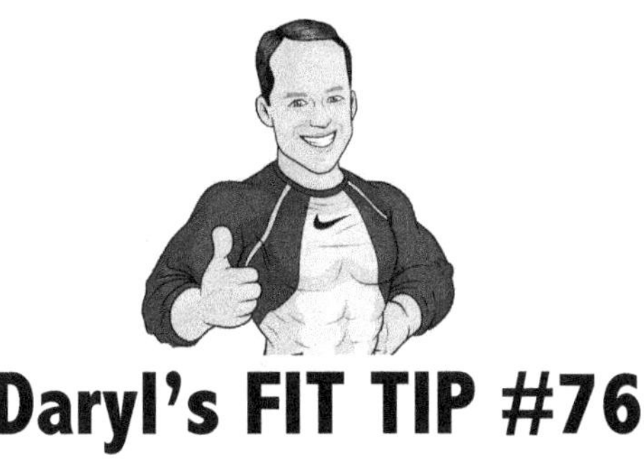

Daryl's FIT TIP #76

AGING

What is aging? Aging is the diminishing number of cells and the shutting down of receptor sites on the cells. From birth to around 25 years old the body is in an anabolic state. The cell number increases and is most abundant. Then after 25 years old the body begins to decline into the catabolic state, losing cells. Over the years as the cell number decreases protein suspension also breaks down. The physical appearance of the body changes, i.e., skin cells decrease making the skin wrinkle and lose elasticity. Inside the body, the cells decrease and shrink. The receptor sites on the cells begin to turn off reducing cellular power and hormonal connections. Glands secrete less hormones, especially the anabolic hormones. Essentially the body is slowly breaking down and dying.

This is the aging process. As depressing as this is there is a way to slow down the aging process== exercise and eat healthy foods.

To really reduce the aging effect it is essential to stay consistent to regular exercise and healthy eating. Irregular exercise and eating only one spear of broccoli a month will not reduce the aging effect. You have to work diligently every week adhering to a regular routine of exercise and healthy eating to make a difference in your cellular make up. Though we can't stop aging completely you can, however, dramatically reduce aging to keep the cells active for much longer than if you live a sedentary life. The cells react to the stimulus that is being presented on the nervous system. If the cells are not being used then they will die off and will not be regenerated because there is no need for more cells. The body WAS DESIGNED TO MOVE AND WORK. The body is it's own generator, when it moves it creates more energy. The more energy that is generated the more cells are activated. The more cells activated the longer mitosis and meiosis lasts allowing for greater protein suspension-- anti-aging.

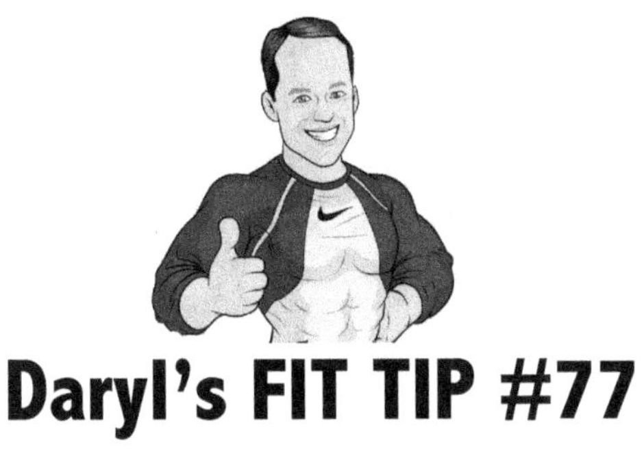

Daryl's FIT TIP #77

THE CURE FOR CANCER

Even though I think it is great that certain foundations all over the country raise billions of dollars a year for cancer research in hopes for a cure, I feel that these efforts are fruitless. All the money raised provides false hope to those who are suffering from cancer.

I said this 20 years in a lecture and the audience thought I had lost my mind, but now it has come to fruition and I still stand firm on my allegation. I said, "the cause for most cancers is right under our noses in the food we eat." However, the research being done is for trying to figure out ways to resolve disease caused by the toxic compounds that are in our food supply without removing the poisons from our food. The money is not used to help create natural ways to decontaminate our food supply. IT'S THE CHEMICALS in our food, and CHEMICALS in the ENVIRONMENT that has increased the risk of cancer.

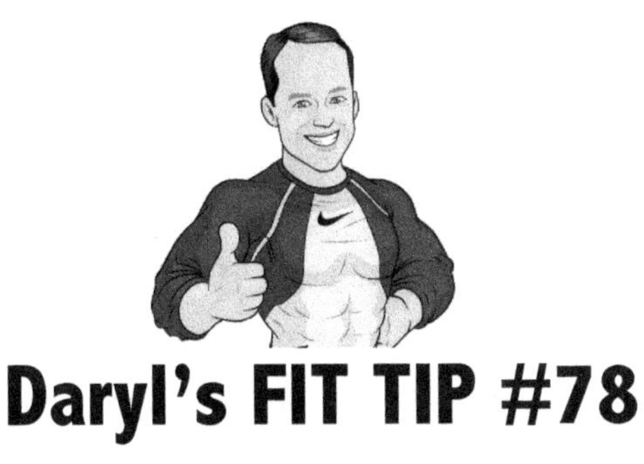

Daryl's FIT TIP #78

NOT FEELING IT

There are some days that I don't feel like training super intense. Sometimes my recovery is hampered and I wake up still feeling tired and worn out from the day before. When the body is not fully restored it is important to NOT over-train. For times like these, I will cut my workout in half using less intensity. It is important to still train but not overdo it. Trying to push yourself through an unrestored body will only make matters worse weakening your body, increase the risk for injury, and ultimately causing a loss in gains.

It is important to listen to your body and to train accordingly.

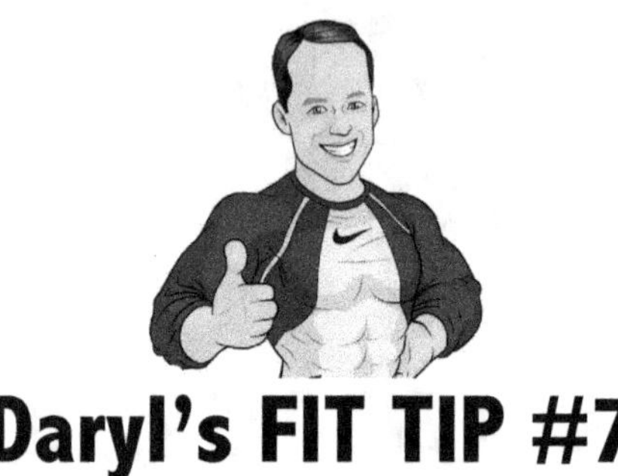

Daryl's FIT TIP #79

UP YOUR PROTEIN

If you exercise you have to consume more protein than if you were sedentary. Exercise breaks down protein of the body. Complete proteins consumed from food helps repair the damaged protein. Some of the benefits of exercise are: capillary expansion, muscle hypertrophy, and increased size and number of enzymes. Increasing the activity and size of the cells requires more protein. You always want to try to maintain a net gain of protein to keep up with the cellular demand and expansion. Falling into a net loss of protein will hinder cellular progress.

Many folks fall into the trap of muscle wasting, where they exercise, tear down tissue, and don't take in enough protein to rebuild, resynthesize, and restore the tissue.

The protein then has to come from their own muscle to feed muscle. This is counterproductive if the protein to repair damaged tissue comes from your own muscles this produces a loss of muscle tissue, and that is something you don't want to happen if you are trying to improve your health and longevity.

Also, remember that the protein necessary to rebuild muscle tissue must be COMPLETE proteins.

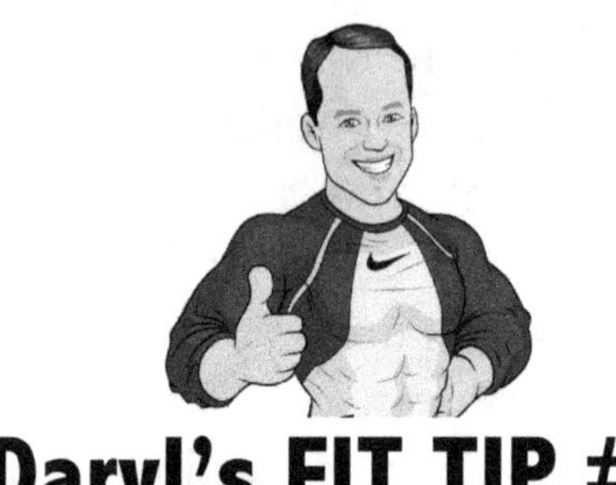

Daryl's FIT TIP #80

INSULIN RESISTANT

Do you suffer from the following?
* Anxiety
* Tired after eating meals
* Fatigued
* Food cravings (especially sugary foods)
* Belly fat
* Not satisfied after meals
* Poor memory and mental focus
* Bladder issues
* Moody, irrational, easily annoyed
* Need caffeine to wake up

If you do then you might be insulin resistant, which means that your pancreas secretes insulin but the cells receptors are blocked or inhibited not allowing insulin to connect and open up the cells, therefore causing an increase in blood sugar, which will end up being stored in fat cells.

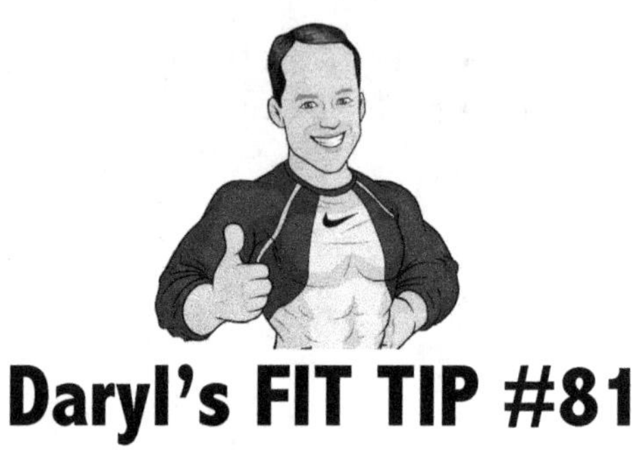

Daryl's FIT TIP #81

Breathe

Step one: Inhale

Step two: Exhale

Repeat often

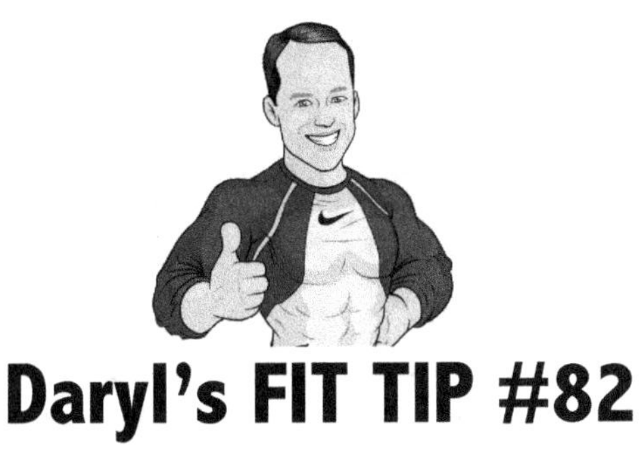

Daryl's FIT TIP #82

SUMMER SNACK

For a cool snack on a WICKED HOT and HUMID day try this. Plain organic yogurt, organic pesticide-free natural blueberries, and walnuts. It's a WICKED good combination. You could even sprinkle a little 90% Organic dark chocolate on the top. Try it today, you will LOVE it!

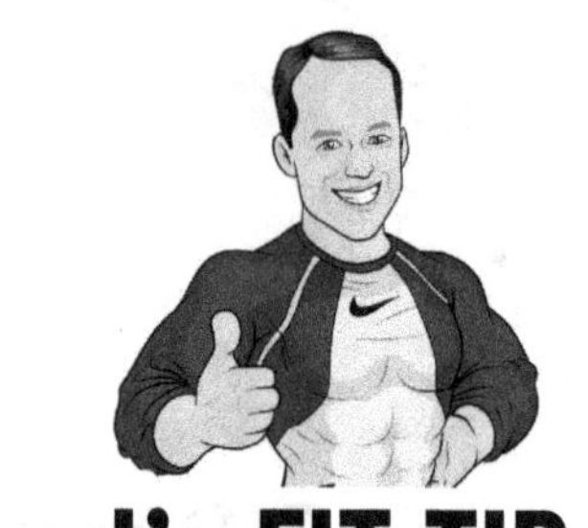

Daryl's FIT TIP #83

LOVE THE BODY YOU ARE IN

So many folks are too hard on themselves. They never seem to be content with the way their body looks. Their mantra is "if I can just lose more weight my life will be better." They end up becoming obsessed with their body. Every thought is directed toward how they look. They can't walk past a mirror without criticizing their own appearance. They are consumed with themselves and can't seem to focus on anything else besides trying to lose weight. They don't like the way they look and it affects their entire being. They could spend their entire life hating their body.

It is important to not take yourself so seriously and to LOVE the body you are in. Accept your limitations and improve upon your strengths. Life is so fragile and precious.

There is so much to enjoy without having to be enslaved into a limited expectation of yourself.

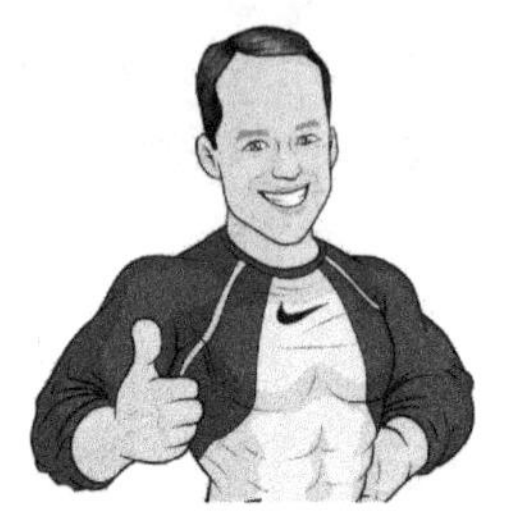

Daryl's FIT TIP #84

GRACE UNDER (blood) PRESSURE

Arteries disperse blood from your heart to every single body part. Blood pressure is the measure of how well all that blood can travel through them. Imbalance of blood pressure can be life-threatening. Extreme low blood pressure is dangerous because of poor oxygen and blood flow to the brain and vital organs.

High blood pressure means that the heart has to pump harder and faster to get the blood delivered throughout the body due to stress factors being presented in the cardiorespiratory system (sympathetic response, blocked artery, obesity, etc...)

Here are 7 steps to keeping your blood pressure in check:

1. Cut out unnecessary salt for your diet.

2. Watch your mid-section. Visceral fat and abdominal fat increase the risk of heart attacks due to the strain that the fat puts on the vital organs.

3. Regular exercise. Exercise can help improve all the systems of the body and help strengthen the cardiovascular system.

4. Eat plenty of potassium. A person needs 4700mg of potassium a day. Potassium helps control sodium levels.

5. Reduce distress. Chronic negative stress wears down the body forcing the heart to work harder and faster increasing the risk of a heart attack.

6. Don't smoke-- ever!

7. Avoid overtraining. Too much physical exertion without proper recovery weakens the cardiovascular system and immune system, which could increase blood pressure.

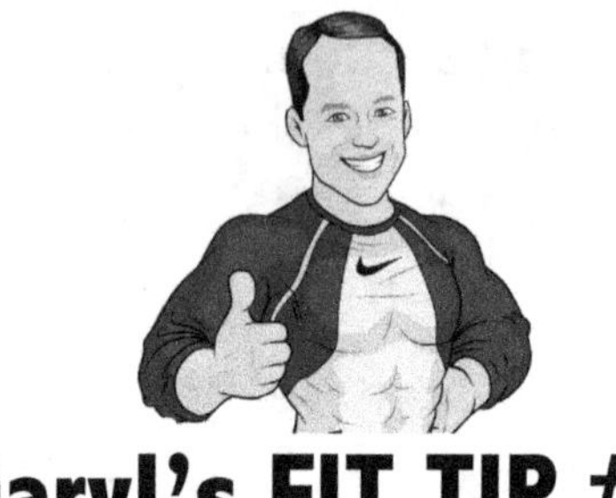

Daryl's FIT TIP #85

CHOLESTEROL

So many people believe that cholesterol is BAD FOR THE BODY. I hate to break it to you but this is WRONG! Cholesterol is essential for the body and vital to your health. It is amazing to me how many people are taking drugs to lower their cholesterol-- it's absurd!

Did you know that the body (liver) makes up to 3000 mg of cholesterol per day, regardless if you cut it out from your diet? The more cholesterol you eat the less your body makes. The body has a keen way of keeping cholesterol balance in the body. So what about HIGH cholesterol? Just because a person has high cholesterol doesn't really mean much. It is believed that a person with high cholesterol has a higher risk of developing a heart attack or stroke. Well, this is not entirely true. If a person is healthy, eating right, and exercising they could have a higher cholesterol reading because they are tearing down muscle, have greater sympathetic nervous system tone, have a better fat and sugar burning system, and have a higher need for hormones, cholesterol is needed for all these changes.

If a person is in poor health and suffers from arteriosclerosis, fatty liver, insulin resistance, adrenal exhaustion, or suffers from chronic stress-related issues will also have high cholesterol. Most of the time these folks are running off a sugar metabolism. The SUGAR is what causes the heart attacks, inflammation, insulin resistance, fatty liver, digestive inflammation, heart disease -- NOT CHOLESTEROL. Cholesterol increases because it is trying to fix the sugar damage in the body.

Healthy foods with natural cholesterol are essential for GOOD HEALTH.

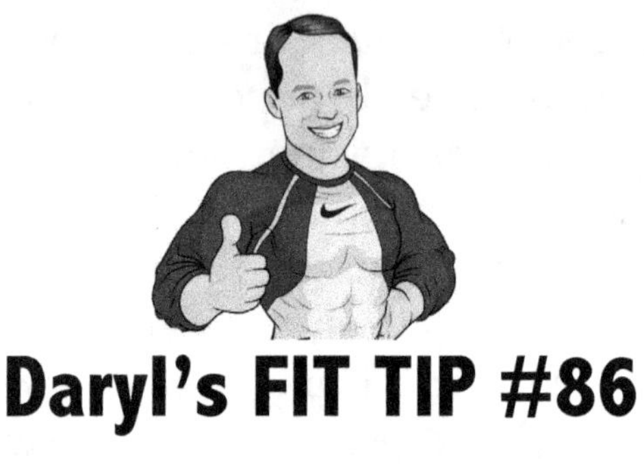

Daryl's FIT TIP #86

SETS and REPS

When weight training it is important to perform enough stimulation to produce a greater anaerobic threshold of the target muscle. In order to challenge the muscle, it is necessary to perform sets and reps. A set constitutes the consecutive execution of a predetermined number of exercise repetitions. Repetitions are how many times the exercise is performed.

The more advanced a person becomes with training the more sets and reps they need to perform to establish greater stimulation on the muscle to increase threshold.

During the first 1-2 sets the exercise might seem easy, this is because the person's neuromuscular threshold has been developed well enough to handle the intensity-- this is when the muscle is "fit." However, progressing further into more sets will challenge the force production of the muscle cells stressing the anaerobic system. The higher the intensity the faster the anaerobic threshold is achieved. In order to develop new growth patterns, force production must exceed the anaerobic threshold. This must be done in a gradual fashion through sets and reps. Working in the high-intensity zone all the time is not conducive. When pushing beyond the anaerobic threshold proper restoration is necessary to rebuild the cellular machinery. Failure to restore properly will result in poor gains.

Here are some physiological adaptations that occur during different set and rep schemes:

Sets: 1-8, Reps: 1-10 Myofibrillar hypertrophy, increased growth hormone production, anaerobic power, increased muscular size

3-6 sets of 12-20 reps: Sarcoplasmic hypertrophy, capillary expansion, greater oxygen capacity, increased testosterone production, increased muscular definition

Whatever your goals remember to always push yourself to establish a new anaerobic threshold. Once the muscle becomes adapted to the stress it becomes complacent and no new effects take place. You essentially just become "fit" at that level.

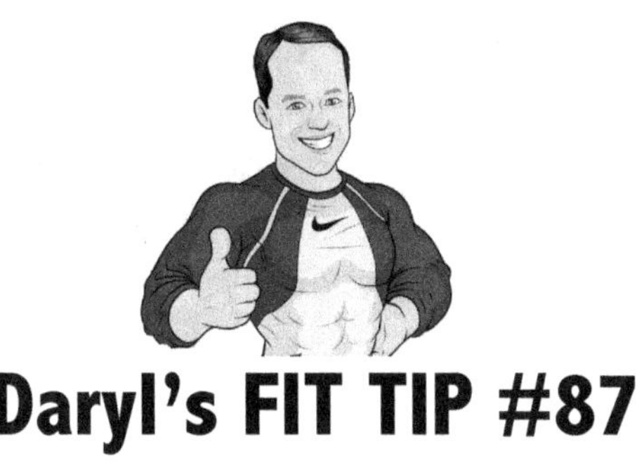

Daryl's FIT TIP #87

CHANGE YOUR SHOES

Sometimes when that nagging back pain starts to develop fixing it might be as simple as buying a new pair of shoes. I have noticed that when I am on my feet for long periods of time for weeks on end I start to develop stiffness and soreness in my lower back. Then, I realize that the shoes I have been wearing have lost their cushioning support. The moment I put on a new pair of well-supported shoes the lower back soreness immediately goes away.

Sneakers have a certain support expectancy and should be tossed out after so many miles in them. Running, walking, or standing for many hours a month will wear down the soles and cushioned support structure reducing the force absorptive properties.

So, if you have started to develop low back stiffness for no apparent reason you might want to evaluate your shoe situation and determine if it is time for a new pair. Doing so might just resolve that nagging pain in the back.

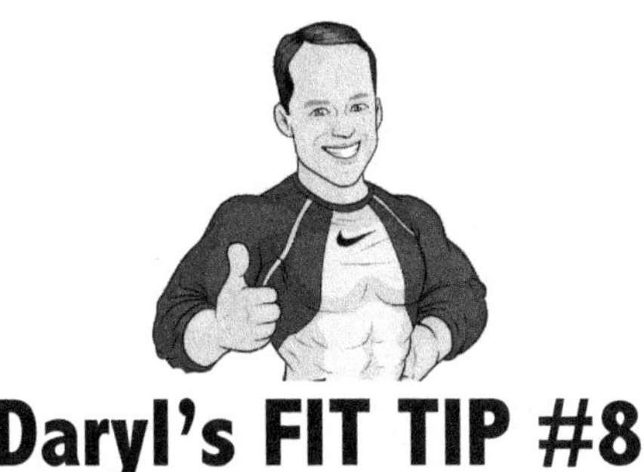

Daryl's FIT TIP #88

ALL TOGETHER NOW

Studies have shown that exercise performed in a group or with a personal trainer-- such as playing a team sport or taking part in an exercise class, or being trained one-on-on-- promotes the production of oxytocin, the hormone commonly held responsible for bonding with others. Some evidence has shown close friendships lead to a lower risk of heart problems, so take advantage of your gym's group classes and personal training and feel the "happy" hormone flow through you-- energizing the systems of your body.

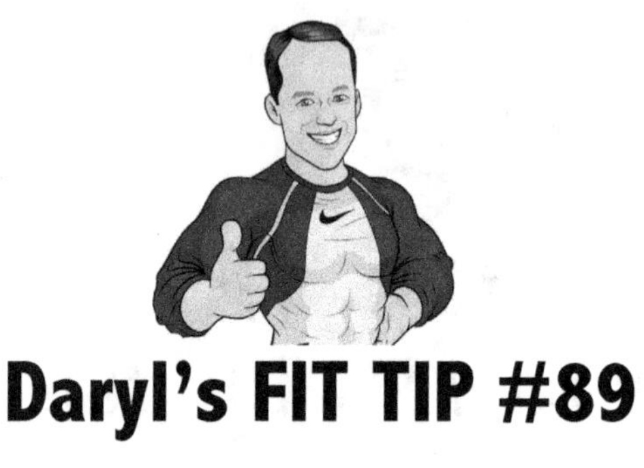

Daryl's FIT TIP #89

CALORIE THINKING

I can't stress it enough YOU CAN'T EAT A CALORIE!!! A calorie is a measurement of heat production. In all my years of teaching nutrition, I have NEVER seen a calorie.

A client came in to me awhile back and said that their doctor said that they needed to eat 1500 calories per day to be healthy and to help control her body weight. When I asked her if she knew what a calorie was, she said that it was food. This is the problem, people associate a calorie as food-- this is wrongful thinking. I asked her how many required daily nutrients (protein, fats, carbs) did the doctor recommend for her. She said the doctor never said anything about nutrients. He said that all she had to do was to eat 1500 calories per day.

So I wrote her up a basic meal plan based on nutrient density which equated to the silly calorie concept (in the picture on the right side). She came in today VERY UPSET because she had gained 10 pounds. I was stunned and asked her if she truly followed the meal plan I prescribed for her. She said, "well NO I didn't, I changed it up to foods I enjoy eating (her daily intake is on the left side of the picture). She was correct in the fact that what she ate equaled to the 1500 calorie idea. However, everything she ate contributed to sugar metabolism releasing a constant flow of insulin throughout the day. All the excess sugar got stored into fat cells, which is why she gained weight. This is why the calorie idea doesn't work. The plan I designed for her was loaded with nutrient-dense foods that would actually help her manage her weight and feed the systems of the body. I explained to her about nutrient intake rather than calorie thinking. Hopefully, this time she will follow the plan.

Counting calories is absolutely RIDICULOUS and serves no purpose. It is important to count the amount of nutrients that your body needs on a daily basis to sustain its physiological demand.

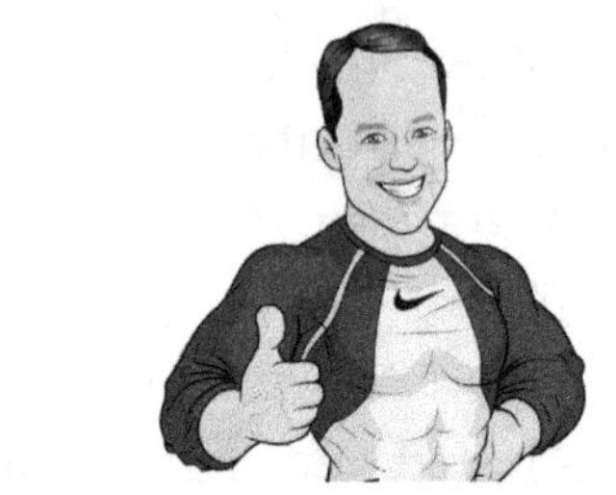

Daryl's FIT TIP #90

MUSCLE BLAST

Here is a little trick of mine to blast the muscles into new stimulation. Perform 1 rep then rest for 6 seconds, then perform 2 reps then rest for 6 seconds, then perform 3 reps rest for 6 seconds. Continue this pattern until you have achieved 10 reps. Use a weight that is about 85% your maximum. This might seem easy but it is very difficult, especially in the latter stages. Give it a try in your workout. It can be done with any exercise. Also, one set is all you will need per exercise using this method.

1 Set:
1 rep, rest 6 seconds
2 reps, rest 6 seconds
3 reps, rest 6 seconds
4 reps, rest 6 seconds

5 reps, rest 6 seconds
6 reps, rest 6 seconds
7 reps, rest 6 seconds
8 reps, rest 6 seconds
9 reps, rest 6 seconds
10 reps, rest 6 seconds

IT'S GONNA BURN those muscles, but it's GONNA FEEL REAL GOOD!!!

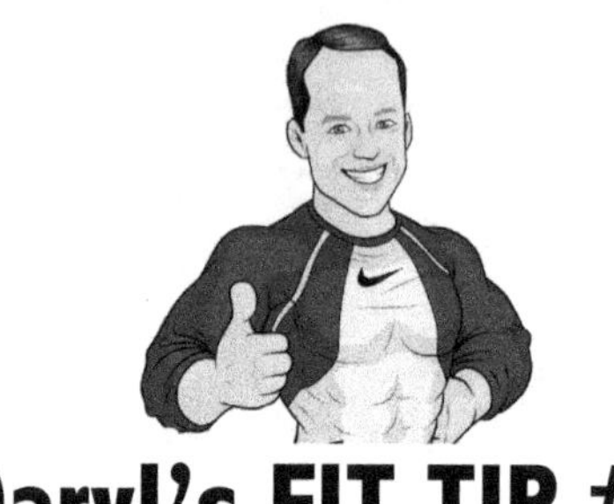

Daryl's FIT TIP #91

BAD COMBINATION

If you are carrying extra body fat around the abdominals or feel horrible after eating a meal you could be eating incorrectly. Never mix concentrated carbohydrates with concentrated proteins, this will result in digestive stress. Gas, bloating, cramps, nausea, increased heart rate, and diarrhea are all symptoms of digestive stress.

Both forms of nutrients digest in different acid/alkaline mediums, and both are dehydrating compounds that require more water to digest efficiently. When they get mixed in the stomach they don't get broken down effectively forming into a thick material chyme that ferments in the intestines causing high levels of nitrogen and strains the water supply. Nitrogen is a gas. So, naturally gas is one of the discomforts that is experienced after eating poorly combined foods. When the digestive tract is stressed cortisol is released to help flush out the digestive tract. This will usually result in loose bowel movements or diarrhea.

In my seminars, I discuss this issue in greater detail and teach the proper methods for cooking and eating nutrient-dense foods in the right combinations.

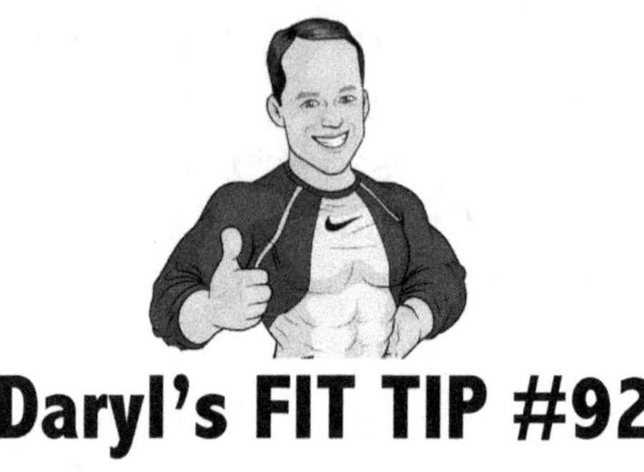

Daryl's FIT TIP #92

BE IT

So many folks talk about it and think about it but never do it. You are either committed to it or not. To BE IT you must live it. Every part of your being must be involved to be what you want to be. IF you want better health you must be willing to commit to it 100% for the rest of your life. What you become is a result of how you live. If you are constantly negative, sick, tired, achy, eat poorly, depend on medications to live, and depressed etc... then you become a negative, sick, tired, achy, depressed person who eats poorly and lives on medications for the rest of your life. If this is the way you want to live your life that is your prerogative.

When it comes to being positive, healthy and fit it takes a commitment for life and discipline. The continuous cycling of stopping and starting an exercise program and eating healthy doesn't work. You are either in or out. In order to keep the systems of the body healthy, it must be challenged on a regular basis. Putting certain food in your body that serves absolutely no purpose is pointless if you are truly committed to being a better YOU!

So many people resort to all the scams and "easy" way schemes to try and cheat the system of eating REAL FOOD and putting in the exercise work. 95% of these people FAIL at achieving better health and changing the way their body looks.

I have heard about all the quick fix remedies, pills, drinks, and hype. I find most of these concoctions useless. The NUMBER ONE trick to better health and longevity is BEING DISCIPLINED to eating REAL FOOD and EXERCISING CORRECTLY and NEVER pollute your system with JUNK food. It's just that simple folks. To BE IT you must LIVE IT!!!

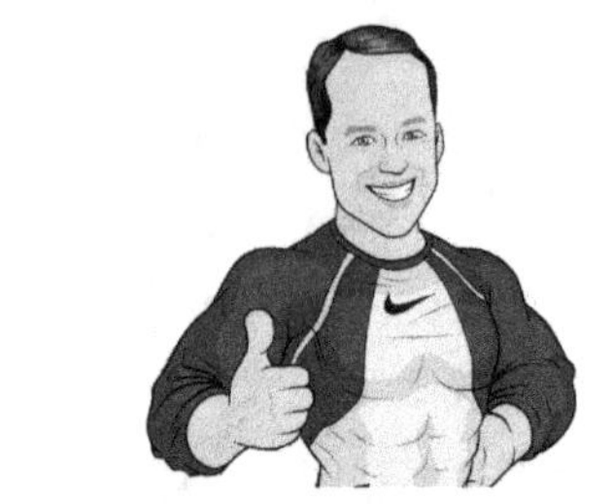

Daryl's FIT TIP #93

DIETING

Dieting is NOT effective in controlling weight; it has NEVER worked, and it NEVER will. Admittedly, you can get temporary weight loss with a diet, but each scheme ultimately gives way to WEIGHT GAIN, and subsequent losses become increasingly difficult. You become hungrier and more obsessed with food, frequently eating out of control. You get TIRED and WEAK, have poor endurance, and generally feel awful about yourself; worst of all you get progressively FATTER on less and less food.

Dieting actually makes you fatter! The whole concept of dieting to lose weight is based on wrongheaded concepts.

The TRUTH is that excess body fat has relatively little to do with the amount of food eaten. Instead, it seems clear that body fat is actually regulated by a control center in the brain referred to as the WEIGHT-REGULATING MECHANISM, which actually "chooses" the amount of body fat that it considers ideal for our needs and then works tirelessly to defend that level. This fat level that the weight-regulating mechanism chooses is called the "setpoint."

Messing up your metabolism by following ridiculous diets will distort your setpoint making you fat.

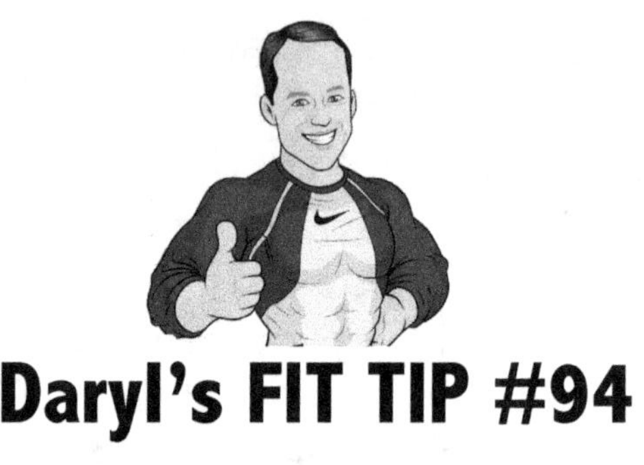

Daryl's FIT TIP #94

6 DEEP BREATHS

A great way to saturate the muscle with oxygen prior to performing the exercise is to take 6 deep breaths. The reason for resting between sets is to re-establish oxygen flow to the muscle. When you lift weights you reduce oxygen to the muscle producing lactic acid build up. The rest period helps clear out the lactic acid to allow oxygen back into the muscle.

Also, taking 6 breaths will reduce wasting energy by sitting around in between sets. It helps you stay focused and keeps the blood volume high in the muscle providing a greater pump. In addition, quick workouts employing short rest periods will increase the overall fat burning effect.

I believe that every second in the weight room should be of value, NEVER waste time during your training session. Every second and every breath counts.

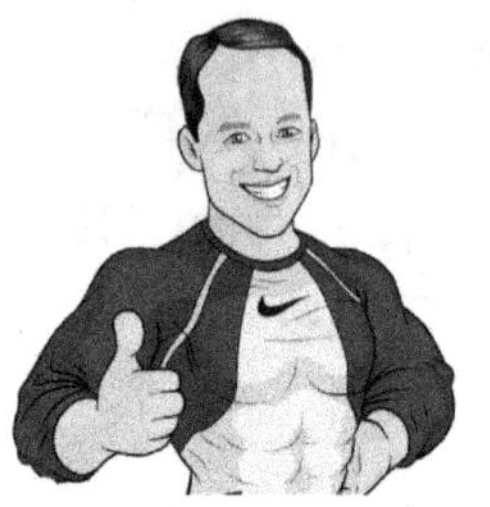

Daryl's FIT TIP #95

IT TAKES TIME TO INCREASE ENZYMES

The muscle machinery must be developed through the correct physiological pathways to increase the power and efficiency of the fat burning enzymes. This process can take several months or even years to reach its fullest capacity. But once the cellular machinery is working at full capacity, fat metabolism can be much more efficient.

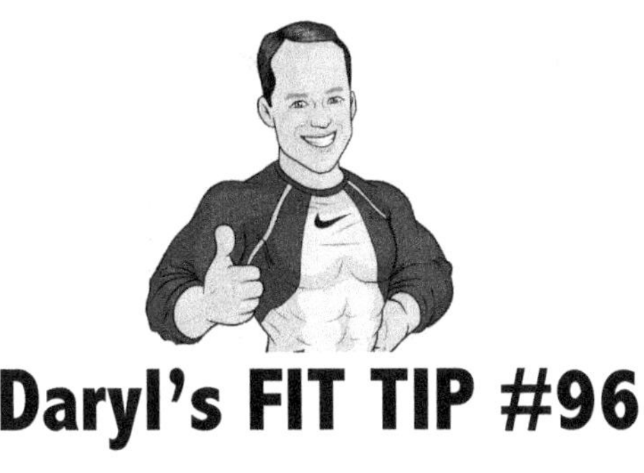

Daryl's FIT TIP #96

6 PACK ABS

well-defined abdominals is the showpiece to a good looking physique. It is believed that if a person performs a countless number of reps and sets working the abdominals that they will get 6-pack abs, however, this is not the case. Yes, it is important to work the abdominals with the correct exercises, but the exercises are only 15% of the equation. Diet makes up the other 85%. When I am often asked the question, "how do I get 6-pack abs?" I say, eat lots of nutrient-dense hearty vegetables. The person then looks at me with a perplexed look thinking that I have lost my mind.

The more nutrient-dense the vegetable the harder the intestines have to work to break down the nutrients. The intestine is made up of smooth muscle tissue. When working hard to extract nutrients the intestines contract to push the food through the system. The more nutrient-dense the food the longer the intestines are contracting. Just by eating hearty vegetables you are essentially working the abdominals for hours after. It takes energy to break down food in the intestines. So you are burning more calories, which will ultimately help metabolize more fat. You will notice that your waistline begins to shrinks and the fat around the abdominals fade away, showing more definition of the abdominal muscles.

IF YOU WANT WELL-DEFINED ABDOMINALS EAT 7-10 CUPS of HEARTY NUTRIENT-DENSE VEGETABLES PER DAY

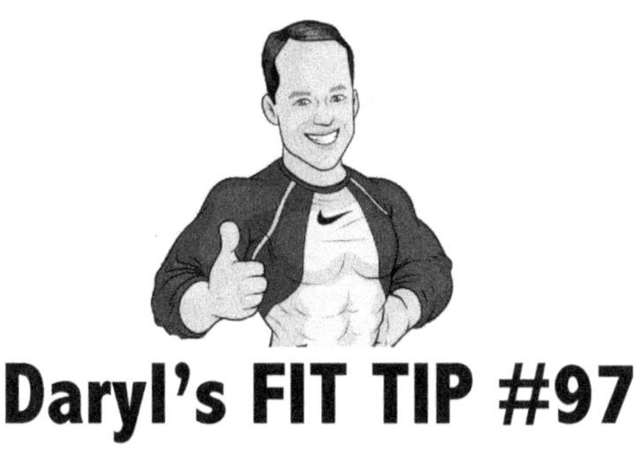

Daryl's FIT TIP #97

WASH YOUR NUTS

If you consume a lot of raw almonds, peanuts, walnuts, etc. This could cause pain in the right side of your body, especially in the right upper neck/scapula region, and can cause digestive distress.

The ducts of the gall-bladder can get blocked as a result of eating too many nuts, which contain phytic acid and lectins. When the gallbladder gets inflamed it triggers the phrenic nerve that runs up the right side of torso and into the neck and head. This is why pain is experienced in the muscles along the nerve root. To avoid this issue, I recommend that you GERMINATE YOUR NUTS.

Soak the nuts in water, 1 tsp. of sea salt, and 1 tsp. of lemon juice. Then put the nuts on a cooking sheet and cook in 150 F oven for 15-

20 minutes. Now you can consume without any adverse effects.

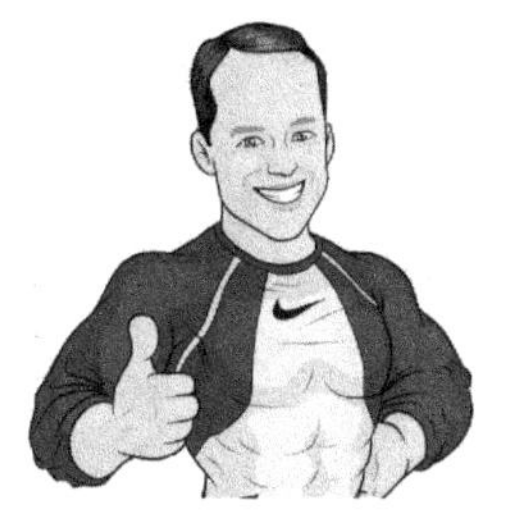

Daryl's FIT TIP #98

The WEIGHT LOSS MISCONCEPTION

ONE of the biggest misconceptions I see in fitness is that PEOPLE THINK THAT IF THEY LOSE WEIGHT THEY ARE HEALTHIER. I hate to break it to you all but the body is NOT designed to LOSE WEIGHT. Here is an image that I put together to illustrate the weight loss misconception. When looking at the before and after picture of this person you immediately notice the loss of weight. You would probably say that she has done a great job and that she is more healthy because she lost weight. WRONG!!!

Even though there was a 20 lb. fat loss, she has lost 30 lbs. of lean body mass in the weight loss process. Her BODY FAT PERCENTAGE didn't change, SHE IS STILL IN THE OBESE category. A high-fat percentage increases risk factors (heart disease, cancer, strokes etc.), NO MATTER WHAT YOUR WEIGHT IS!!!

Losing muscle tissue is the LAST thing you want to do if you are trying to burn fat off your body. It's through muscle metabolism that fat is burned. If you WASTE muscle tissue you LOSE the ability to burn fat. The body perceives the loss of muscle as a threat to the body and will hold on to fat as a defense mechanism.

Commercial nutrition plans that sell "WEIGHT LOSS" programs are scams and should be avoided. A true program is one that promotes FAT LOSS, not weight loss. This is why I DO NOT LIKE WEIGHT WATCHERS and similar programs. These programs help a person lose weight-- that is true. But many times the person loses too much muscle in the process and not enough of the fat. And, will 95% of the time gain all the weight back in the form of fat. You get fatter around the belly, and weight watchers get's fatter in the wallet-- thanks to you!

If you exercise to LOSE WEIGHT then you are doomed to fail. Scales are USELESS!!! Forcing yourself to weigh a certain number is POINTLESS!!! You will only end messing up your metabolism, making it even harder to lose fat.

It ALL COMES DOWN to a healthy body composition. If your fat percentages are in the healthy parameters for your body then whatever your weight is, is what your body is designed to weigh.

If you exercise to be more efficient at burning fat then you will most likely succeed.

STOP WASTING YOUR TIME WITH PROGRAMS AND CONCEPTS THAT PROMOTE WEIGHT LOSS!

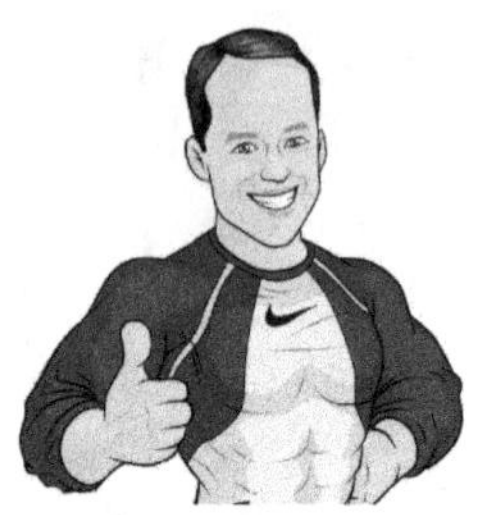

Daryl's FIT TIP #99

WHAT'S THE POINT OF EXERCISE

Though many people don't like it, exercise is the "fountain of youth." The body is designed to move. The body is its own generator. When we move the body gets energized. The POINT to exercise is to control and strengthen the systems of the body. The greatest benefit of exercise is to control the balance and strength of the neuromuscular system (nervous and musculoskeletal system).

Having better parasympathetic and sympathetic nervous system tone is why we exercise. Poor tone results in a low-stress threshold, which can result in the overproduction of stress hormones. These stress hormones can weaken the body, especially the endocrine system, which will result in excess fat gain and inflammation.

Exercise is "CONTROLLED" stress that builds the stress threshold. When the stress threshold is high a person can tolerate physical and emotional stress much better without causing adverse effects to the body systems. Improving parasympathetic and sympathetic tone is the key to being FIT. This is what being "toned" means.

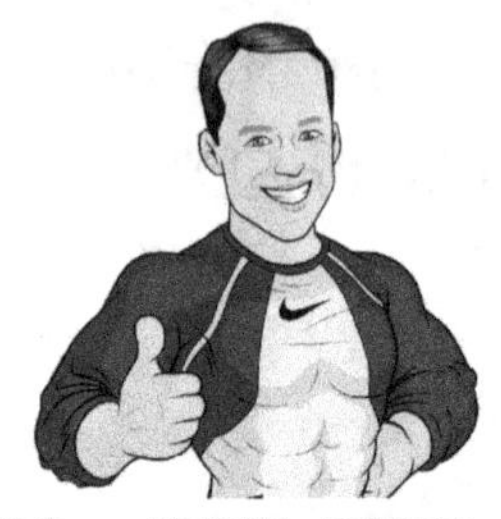

Daryl's FIT TIP #100

OVERTONUS

It is important to establish neural conductivity between muscle cells to enhance contractibility. During a muscle contraction, the neuron activates a sequence of chemicals that elicit the muscle cell to turn on and contract. This process is sensitive to resistance. If the workload is too much then the synaptic transmission becomes weak. The weak signal forces the nervous system to release stress hormones to help stop further damage to the tissue. When the motor units of a muscle cell are overworked they begin to receive only fragments of the neuronal signal. A shaky, weak feeling is felt in the muscle this is known as overtonus. Once this feeling occurs exercise should be stopped. Continuing to exercise will only produce a negative effect and could result in loss of gains, or injury.

Other Books by Daryl

Healthy Living: For a Better YOU! (2017) Fitness and nutrition information can be overwhelming and too complex to comprehend. Healthy Living is an easy to understand approach to the principles of fitness and nutrition. Daryl Conant has simplified the complex concepts of fitness and nutrition to help people understand how the body works in conjunction with improving health. In addition to great information, Healthy Living also contains complete exercise programs to build the body. And as a bonus, Daryl has included his Secrets to Fat Loss; 30 great tips to help you achieve a BETTER YOU...

ConVINCEd: (2017) The sequel to InVINCEable™. Vince Gironda was one of the greatest trainers in bodybuilding history. **ConVINCEd** is an encyclopedia of Vince's true natural body. Includes training theory, research studies of Vince's exercises, and illustrations of 235 of Vince's exercises. It is a must have for anyone interested in True Natural Bodybuilding.

Positopes: *All Things Positive (2016)* Positive energy is the essence of all that is good in this world and universe. Positopes explores positive energy in a whole different perspective. Daryl shares his discoveries about positive energy in this inspiring and enlightening manuscript. We all have the ability to do great things and it all begins with being positive.

CiviLIESationTM: *The Undeniable Truth (2015)* Is an in-depth look at what we are, who we are, and the ultimate purpose of our existence. The Cosmos is a grand miracle and though we don't know its origin or purpose one thing does remain true and that is that the entire Cosmos is made up of energy: the energy of Creation. The earth is a living biosphere that is a product of the atomic expansion of the universe. CiviLIESationTM explores illusionary perceptions, projections, and reflections of the ego. CiviLIESationTM is a presentation of conscious awareness.

Buff Daddy: *Body Building For The Family Man (2011)* Buff Daddy is a complete program for helping the family man stay in great physical condition while in the trenches of parenthood. Being a family man is an honor and takes total unselfish underlying commitment. In order to have a successful marriage a couple must balance their lives in accordance to their families needs, while still taking care of themselves.

Diet Earth: *The Complete Nutrition Solution (2009)* Nutrition is a complex science that can be overwhelming to comprehend. Daryl takes the complexity out of the science of nutrition and presents an easy to follow approach to understanding: how, what, and when to eat, and why we need to eat to maintain good health.

InVINCEeable *The Methods of Vince Gironda (2008)* One of Daryl's greatest influences in bodybuilding was the "Iron Guru" Vince Gironda. Vince was one of the most knowledgeable trainers in the history of fitness. Daryl learned first hand from Vince. After finding out about Vince's death in 1995. Daryl decided to write a book to give tribute to his mentor, explaining many of the techniques that Vince taught.

These publications can be purchased at:

www.darylconant.com

Follow my FIT TIPS on Facebook™

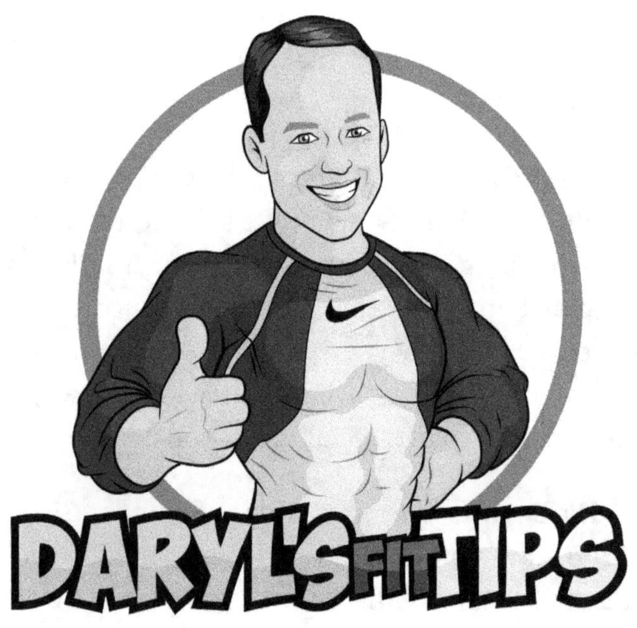

About the Author:

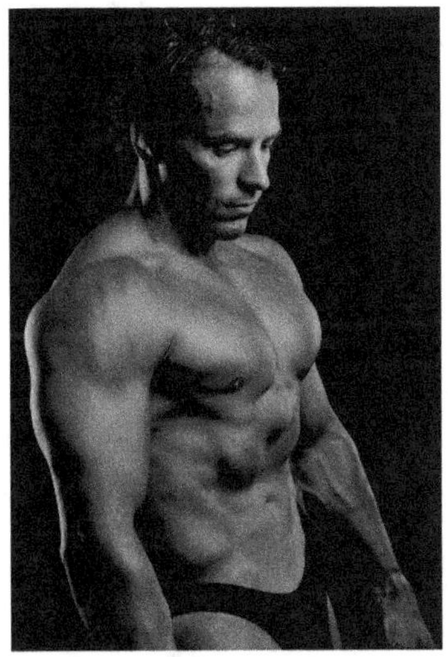

Daryl Conant, M.Ed., is an Author, Exercise Physiologist, Professional Strength Coach, Natural Bodybuilder, Inventor, and owner of Fitness Nut Enterprises, LLC in Kennebunk, Maine. Daryl obtains two Bachelor degrees: in Psychology and Exercise Physiology, and a Master's degree in Exercise Science. He has three wonderful children and a beautiful wife who are his main inspiration for doing great things in this world. Daryl's passion for teaching about nutrition, health, and fitness is insatiable. He loves sharing what he knows with others, so that they too can reap the benefits of good health.

www.ingramcontent.com/pod-product-compliance
Lightning Source LLC
Chambersburg PA
CBHW061800250726
48657CB00001B/220